Professionalism

Key Themes in Health and Social Care series

Nick J. Fox, *The Body*
Janet Hargreaves & Louise Page, *Reflective Practice*

Professionalism

ALAN CRIBB AND SHARON GEWIRTZ

polity

First published in 2015 by Polity Press

Polity Press
65 Bridge Street
Cambridge CB2 1UR, UK

Polity Press
350 Main Street
Malden, MA 02148, USA

ISBN-13: 978-0-7456-5316-7
ISBN-13: 978-0-7456-5317-4 (pb)

A catalogue record for this book is available from the British Library.

Library of Congress Cataloging-in-Publication Data

Cribb, Alan, author.
  Professionalism / Alan Cribb, Sharon Gewirtz.
    p. ; cm.
  Includes bibliographical references and index.
  ISBN 978-0-7456-5316-7 -- ISBN 978-0-7456-5317-4 (pb)
  I. Gewirtz, Sharon, 1964- , author. II. Title.
  [DNLM: 1. Health Occupations. 2. Professional Role. 3. Ethics, Professional. 4. Social Work. W 21]
  R690
  610.69--dc23
                                                            2014043492

Typeset in 10.25/13 Scala by
Servis Filmsetting Limited, Stockport, Cheshire
Printed and bound in the United Kingdom by Clays Ltd, St Ives PLC

For further information on Polity, visit our website: politybooks.com

Contents

Preface

This is, obviously, only one of the many short books about professionalism that could be written. One such book might usefully start by looking at codes of professional practice and reviewing and advocating the standards of behaviour and quality that apply to health and social care practitioners. What is required of practitioners, for example, when it comes to confidentiality, honesty or stewardship of scarce resources? Another book might begin from critiques of professional power and argue that professionalism is no longer a credible notion in contemporary social conditions. The latter text would have a predominantly sceptical, even dismissive, tone.

This book, although it covers similar themes and material, takes neither of these lines. We hope it is an encouraging text and one that might help support the understanding – and exercise – of professionalism. However, it does not take the idea of professionalism for granted. The two broad organizing questions that lie behind the book's arguments are: Is professionalism desirable and is professionalism possible? Taking these questions seriously means not taking all of the social apparatus surrounding professionalism (for example, codes of practice and the professional bodies that issue them) at face value. It means standing back and asking about the visions, ideals and personal virtues that lie behind the language of professionalism, and asking whether or not these visions, ideals and virtues are meaningful and practicable for current health and social care systems and practitioners.

We believe, and will argue, that these questions can be answered in the affirmative. But in order to come to this conclusion, we suggest, it is first necessary to be clear about the many challenges posed by such questions, including the challenges of critics and sceptics. Much of the book's focus is on professional dilemmas, but here our primary interest is not in the specific dilemmas that might face practitioners (for example, those concerning compulsory treatment, euthanasia, allocating budgets, etc.) but rather the fundamental dilemmas of determining what it means to be a professional in current working contexts. In very broad terms, this involves, for example, balancing a traditional emphasis on being an 'autonomous expert' with ever-increasing demands to be responsive and accountable to both service users and managers. Those occupying roles in health and social care operate under immense pressure not only from sheer volume of work but also from this constant need to balance competing perspectives and voices. What can and should professionalism look like under these circumstances?

We start, in chapter 1, by thinking about the image of professionals as socially special, and perhaps particularly admirable, individuals. How does this image connect to the fact that some professionals can do bad things? Our hope is to begin to shed light on how professional status and roles place people in relatively powerful positions – for good or ill. In chapter 2, we consider the idea that the language of professionalism has spread so widely and thinly as to become an empty public relations 'brand', but then go on to look for some core sense of profession that might properly underpin professionalism as an ideal. The difficulty this uncovers is that conceptions of profession and professionalism are not fixed – new versions of professionalism have emerged along with new expectations for health and social care practitioners. We track some of these changing conceptions, contrasting traditional conceptions of professionalism with some versions of 'new professionalism'. In chapter 3, we seriously explore the idea that calls for professionalism are unrealistic – because changing social conditions and expectations make traditional conceptions of professionalism less relevant and because changing working conditions make the delivery of 'new professionalism' practically impossible, even laying aside question marks about its coherence as a version of professionalism. Whilst not accepting the thesis that professionalism is now a practical impossibility, we explore these issues to show just how challenging it is to formulate, practise and socially underpin forms of professionalism in the contemporary workplace.

In the remainder of the book, we set out to respond to these challenges. First, in chapter 4, we map out and illustrate a summary and ideal-type conception of professionalism – as the accomplished exercise of expertise-based social authority – that we think can stretch to serve current practice conditions and that embodies something both desirable and, at least to a degree, possible (albeit demanding) for many practitioners. This conception draws upon the discussions earlier in the book and, we suggest, is general enough to hold together different perspectives on, and versions of, professionalism but needs interpretation and application in contemporary conditions. We then set out to analyse and illustrate the dilemmas involved in both living out (chapter 5) and socially and institutionally supporting (chapter 6) this notion of professionalism. Our argument is that these dilemmas are inherent in professionalism – and that professionalism does not consist in identifying 'what works' so much as in being ready to question and debate what counts as working from case to case. These two chapters thus help to 'fill out' the general account of professionalism offered in chapter 4 for the conditions of contemporary health and social care. The account that emerges is of a 'critically reflexive' professionalism – a professionalism which is continuously negotiated with others and routinely combines relational as well as technical forms of expertise, which is ready to embrace critique and self-doubt, and which draws upon practitioners' humanity and practical wisdom. This conception of professionalism also entails that practitioners will understand their work, and engage with it, with sensitivity towards broader debates about social and civic purposes. In chapter 7, the concluding chapter, we retell the story of the book by returning to the idea of individual practitioners, or at least their role models, as embodying admirable qualities. What kind of identities can and should practitioners aspire to and enact if they want to embody the ideals and virtues of professionalism in their working lives? Our intended audience here, as throughout the book, is practitioners who work in health and social care, but we imagine that the themes and topics we discuss will have many resonances for people working in other professional roles.

This book, in short, explores and reflects upon the complex and disputed territory of professionalism. We hope that it will stimulate readers' own explorations and reflections; indeed, this is the primary aim of the book. Although we do offer arguments and observations of our own about the nature and importance of professional roles and professionalism, we are hoping that readers will approach the book not looking to take away 'answers' but rather to find material to think about. After all, we would suggest, professionalism entails being able to think things through and make judgements for oneself, albeit within frameworks of support provided by others.

Acknowledgements

We would like to thank all our colleagues in the Centre for Public Policy Research, King's College, London for being wonderful people to work with and, more specifically, for many criss-crossing conversations relating to things discussed in this book which we have enjoyed over the years. We are also very grateful to Pat Mahony and Ian Hextall who co-organized an ESRC seminar series on professional identities and education with us which gave us the opportunity to think around the topic of professionalism. Huge thanks go to Vikki Entwistle and John Owens who provided very encouraging and constructive comments on an earlier draft of the book. Alan would also particularly like to thank the Health Foundation for funding which made the writing of this book possible and his colleagues there, including Adrian Sieff, Alf Collins and Nick Barber for support, stimulation and valuable feedback on ideas.

As before, it has been a pleasure to work with Polity Press. Emma Hutchinson and Pascal Porcheron have been patient, helpful and suitably challenging. We are grateful to them and also to the two anonymous reviewers whose comments, along with those from Vikki and John, were invaluable in helping us to complete the manuscript.

CHAPTER ONE

Heroes and Anti-Heroes

Are health and social care professionals, and perhaps other professionals also, somehow special? This is a large – and deliberately vague – question which we will come back to from time to time. But we can begin to respond to it straight away.

There is a sense in which all professionals, including, for example, health professionals, are special because they are just different from one another and from 'non-professionals'. That is, all professionals occupy specific and distinctive social roles – they participate in a division of labour between people and 'specialize' in various areas of work, tasks and goals. If someone collapses in an airport departure lounge – perhaps just fainting with exhaustion, perhaps because of something more serious – it makes sense that it is a doctor or a nurse, rather than an accountant or retail assistant, who rushes across to see what can be done. They are, generally speaking, more likely to have relevant knowledge and experience. They are, for this reason, also more likely to feel confident and comfortable offering this kind of help. In turn, this suggests another sense in which some professionals are arguably special. It is not just that most other bystanders would feel wary of the intrusion entailed by approaching the collapsed individual and their family members and, even more so, by crouching down on the ground, putting their faces in close and reaching out to touch them. It is also that some professionals have a distinctive kind of social licence to be able to 'get up close and personal', and so those on the receiving end of these attentions are also much more likely to feel comfortable and reassured if they know that it is a health or social care professional attending

to them. These considerations about personal space and intimacy are relatively unique to the care professions. (There are
some similarities in the hair and beauty sector, for example,
but the corresponding licence is both more conditional and
more restricted.) However, there are some analogous aspects
to other professions. We may, for example, allow a lawyer or
social worker to 'invade' the intimate details of our finances
but would resist having these shared more widely.

This social licence for 'invasion' and intimacy suggests a
further sense in which care professionals might be seen as
special. When we are approached by a doctor, nurse or social
worker proffering their services, it is normal to assume not
only that they have relevant knowledge but also that they intend
to do some good. The social role of these professionals would
not make sense unless both these presumptions applied – a
presumption of knowledge and also one of beneficence. If all
we knew about someone was that they had insight into human
biology and well-being, but we had no sense of whether they
had an interest in promoting or in positively undermining our
biological, psychological or social well-being, then we would,
of course, be reluctant to let them near us. These professionals
are perhaps therefore 'ethically special'. We can, or at least we
certainly hope we can, take their beneficence for granted. The
same presumption does not apply if we are approached by a
stranger on the street, or if we are approached by a car sales-
person or many other people doing their jobs.

In this chapter, we will explore this notion of specialness
further. In the first half of the chapter, using the example of
doctors and nurses, we will explore the image of some professionals as 'special beings' and both how this can serve
as a source of inspiration and motivation and how such an
image can be abused and provide a cover for wrongdoing. In
the second half of the chapter, we will consider how professions constitute a 'special category' of worker and some of the
forms of hierarchy and social power associated with this. We
will conclude by pointing towards one of the core themes of

the book by asking what, if anything, is special or distinctive about professionalism.

Gods and angels

Some of the best-known images of doctors and nurses seemingly distil the idea of the ethically special agent into something approaching a pure essence of goodness. According to these images, doctors and nurses, as they move amongst us, are a kind of divine presence or at least symbolically represent something of divine love on the human plane. These representations are no doubt rather old-fashioned and, if positively articulated, subject to all kinds of qualifications or objections, but they persist and are culturally influential. There are many other representations that carry similar, albeit less transcendental, connotations of the ethically special, indeed of the ethically extraordinary, health professional. Doctors, nurses and others can be characterized as 'saints', embodying devotion to others and sustained self-sacrifice. They can, in less religious language, be seen as 'heroic' – men or women of exceptional strength of character who embody great and admirable qualities. Even in terms of popular culture, the health professionals who feature as the 'heroes' in television or film dramas, whilst often 'interestingly flawed', are typically exceptional people who display uncommon degrees of conscientiousness and care.

A few historical health professionals have, in certain contexts, been granted iconic status as cultural heroines and heroes, exemplifying goodness in many of these ways – as models of saintliness, beneficence and courage. This is the case, for example, with Florence Nightingale and Albert Schweitzer. These were two giant figures of the nineteenth and twentieth centuries, polymaths whose complex and multi-faceted lives are not summarized easily even in many volumes of biography. However, they also existed as simplified figures in children's storybooks and textbooks, and as household names, standing for the human goodness that can be done by innovation and dedication in health care. They, along with many other figures, thus served as an example and inspiration to generations of people who aspired to become, and make a contribution as, health professionals and who wished to emulate some of the qualities of service represented by these exemplars.

These days, it is commonplace for icons to be torn down and for historical figures to be taken off their pedestals and reappraised. But – leaving that revisionist instinct on one side – it may be worth briefly reminding ourselves of some of the elements of the simplified 'heroic' versions of Nightingale and Schweitzer. Partly, this is because these simplifications do represent one dimension of 'the whole truth' and, partly, because they help to indicate some of the fundamentally important ideals and challenges of health and social care.

Florence Nightingale, for example, determined to give up a life of relative comfort – reflecting the expectations of her class and gender – and to train as a nurse and then, whilst working in London, to give up a role lacking in significant day-to-day threat in order to travel to Crimea and confront, and to some degree share, the dreadful circumstances of the soldiers who, in addition to their wounds, were risking death from cholera and malaria and being cared for in an ill-equipped and ill-resourced army hospital. It is difficult to overstate the difference that the presence of Nightingale and the other nurses could make to this situation. In a sense, the idea of 'presence' indicates a fundamental part of the difference – men who might otherwise have felt completely abandoned had people around them focused upon them and their needs. In turn, this means, of course, being in a position to provide immediate practical help and care. In addition, however, for Nightingale there was the possibility of more structural and strategic action, and of developing what is nowadays often called an 'advocacy' role – to both work and campaign for better sanitation and nutrition in army hospitals and for better training for army medical and nursing staff to underpin more effective care. Furthermore, Nightingale took on a 'research role', applying her knowledge of statistics to wounds, disease transmission and death in hospitals, thereby making a yet broader contribution to epidemiology and public health. These advocacy, education and research roles entailed confrontation with the existing establishment of army medicine and health care more generally and could not have been accomplished without a good deal of personal resilience and courage.

Like Nightingale, Albert Schweitzer had a powerful sense of 'calling'. Although he had many accomplishments, he is perhaps best known for his medical missionary work in what is now Gabon (formerly French Equatorial Africa) where he established a hospital at Lambaréné. Schweitzer was a successful musician and theologian whose quest to be a medical missionary necessitated him standing back from these successes to embark on seven years of medical training at the age of thirty. Although motivated by his faith, his mission also entailed a lot of hard physical work – in the first instance, creating a clearing in the jungle and working on the construction of the first small buildings. By the time of his death aged 90 in Lambaréné in 1965, it was a well-established health facility with 350 beds in addition to a leper colony, and he himself had operated upon and cared for thousands of local people. The challenges posed by the very hot climate, the local disease burden and the very restricted resources were formidable. Although Schweitzer had his critics, there can be no doubting the extraordinary challenges he had to overcome to enact his missionary work or the substantial numbers of people who benefited from the work of the hospital. For that reason, and his preparedness to live a life without an emphasis on material possessions (allied perhaps to his influential teachings on 'Reverence for Life'), many people have viewed him as both a modern saint and a practical hero.

It is important to acknowledge that there is something odd about starting a book on professionalism with Nightingale and Schweitzer. First, these were clearly unique and extraordinary human beings. Any treatment of professionalism must ultimately relate to what might reasonably be expected of the relatively large numbers of people who make up professional groups. Second, given the groundbreaking nature of the work they did, these two historical figures, whilst broadly belonging to the traditions and occupations of nursing and medicine respectively, are arguably not best understood as 'members of professions' in the same way that contemporary nurses and doctors are, but rather as pioneers and exceptions.

However, as we have indicated, there is also something fitting about starting with icons such as these. At least at a symbolic level, reference to such figures helps to conjure up and convey some of the ideals (and idealizations) reflected in the image of 'ethically special' health and social care professionals. When it comes to dispositions such as dedication, or altruism, or self-sacrifice, for example, 'ordinary' professionals may feel that they have more modest claims to make. But they may nonetheless aspire to such dispositions and see them as an important part of their personal and professional identity. The inspiring individuals they encounter in their everyday training and practice, and stories about more or less distant role models, all help to give shape to professional ideals and visions. And this need not be viewed as some 'airy-fairy' fancy. It is arguable that one of the most important functions of professional roles is that they can provide a real-world framework in which people can develop and enact ethically worthwhile dispositions. To become a nurse, doctor or social worker, for example, means – whatever else – to be given the opportunity to do valuable things for others and to develop the knowledge and dispositions – the intellectual and ethical 'virtues' – to translate that aspiration into something practical. Many of the characteristics of professional groups and bodies – relating to entry, standard setting, ethical codes and accountability structures, for example, have the avowed rationale of promoting and protecting this possibility.

Professional roles can enable people to do good. We do not want to lose sight of this simple but important idea in this book. Indeed, we wish to stress this idea and to do our best to defend its importance. But there is a problem with this simple idea that needs to be acknowledged straight away. The problem is manifest in the fact that we have talked both about the 'image' of professionals as 'ethically special' and also about the potential for 'ethically special' practice. Whenever ethics is talked about, there is the constant danger that what is in question is actually image rather than substance, 'public relations' rather than practice. And images and PR can disguise realities as well as reveal them. A blunt way of stating the potential problem here is to note the fact that *professional roles can also enable people to do 'bad' (i.e. harm or wrong)*.

Murderers and demons

Professionals sometimes do bad things – they can be straightforwardly corrupt, or fail to follow professional ethics guidelines or neglect their clients in various ways. There are countless mundane wrongdoings that might be reviewed here. But in this section we want to reflect a little on some more extreme cases. We want to pause and think about the fact that some health professionals, for example, have done some utterly dreadful things. This means turning our attention away from celebrated icons and towards icons of notoriety. There are a number of cases that could be discussed in this context, including the involvement of professionals in awful research scandals and even in genocidal atrocities. But we will instead confine ourselves to cases of health professionals as 'serial killers', and in particular to the cases of Beverly Allitt and Harold Shipman.

Beverly Allitt worked for a short time as a nurse in the UK National Health Service (NHS). Following a six-month contract, in 1991 on the children's ward of Grantham General Hospital, Allitt was convicted of murdering four children and seriously injuring (and in some cases attempting to murder) nine other children. Allitt used large doses of insulin to kill her victims. She was sentenced to thirteen concurrent terms of life imprisonment. Clearly, these facts were utterly devastating ones for the families affected, but they also had considerable impact for the institutions concerned and for the broader nursing profession and wider society. The popular media soon labelled Allitt as 'the Angel of Death'. As is typical with serial killers, she was also branded as a 'monster' and as 'evil'. As is also typical, there was much speculation around the axis of whether the perpetrator of such dark offences was 'mad' rather than 'bad'. In this instance, the official consensus was that Allitt was herself seriously unwell. She was judged to have severe mental health problems (possibly including some indications of Munchausen Syndrome by Proxy) and detained in a maximum security hospital. Of course, an important component of the alarm and horror surrounding the Allitt case was the fact that someone working as a nurse – and charged, in this case, with looking after other people's children – could be capable of such crimes. This horror was compounded by media accounts of how Allitt befriended the parents of her victims and thereby encouraged their trust in her.

There are some parallels between the Allitt case and that of Harold Shipman but also very many divergences. Shipman was a British doctor who worked for many years as a general practitioner (GP) in the NHS. Unlike Allitt, he had firmly established a place for himself within the UK health service, had experienced a long career as a working professional and was regarded by many of his patients as a good doctor. The scale of his killings was also correspondingly (and staggeringly) large. He was judged, by an inquiry into his case, to have killed 240 patients, ten when working as a junior hospital doctor, but most of them whilst working in the community as a 'family doctor' in Yorkshire and Greater Manchester in the North of England. Shipman killed a range of people over his career but his typical victims were older people (especially women over 75 years of age). He would visit patients of his in their own homes, administer lethal injections of diamorphine and then falsify death certificates to indicate some other underlying cause of death. Shipman hanged himself in a prison cell four years after his conviction in 2000 for the murder of fifteen of his victims, for which he was sentenced to fifteen consecutive terms of life imprisonment.

Unsurprisingly, both Allitt and Shipman were sometimes represented in popular media as 'devils' or 'demons', virtually the opposite of the connotations of divinity that, as we have seen, are more often deployed in the case of health professionals. They are certainly, as we should stress again, 'extreme' and exceptional cases. So why discuss them in a book about professionalism? What is their possible relevance to 'ordinary' professionals? Their relevance is not, of course, that we should go around suspecting other professionals of being capable of equivalent crimes. Rather, the point of considering these extreme cases is to draw attention to the way that membership of professional roles can both create, and mask, opportunities for causing harm and doing wrong. These opportunities are created because such roles enable people to gain 'privileged access' to others, for example, to their hospital bedsides and to their front rooms, including, in these cases, being allowed to administer injections. These opportunities are masked because the fact that someone is occupying a professional role grants them a considerable degree of social and interpersonal legitimacy. There is a general presumption that people in certain roles are trustworthy and there are further chances for them to actively cultivate and trade on trust with individuals, chances that both Allitt and Shipman exploited in a dreadful way.

Indeed, we would argue that there is a danger in not considering these cases, and in pushing them to the margins on the assertion that they are wholly, purely and simply exceptional, with absolutely no relevance for the vast majority of 'normal', broadly well-intentioned and responsible practitioners. The tendency to marginalize such cases is, of course, reinforced by designations such as 'monster' or by reference to 'evil'. Labels such as these can act as 'thought-stoppers', and there are two risks attached to this. First, it can make us neglect the fact that there may be some parallels worth exploring, however minimal, between these outlying cases and some more typical cases, and we will come back to this possibility shortly. Second, by focusing on the (exceptional) characteristics of the individuals concerned, it can stop us from thinking about the broader contexts and the more structural lessons such cases can teach – such as the one we are stressing here, the 'masking' potential of professional roles. To reiterate, the crucial point is that the idea of the 'ethically special' professional cuts both ways – professional roles can serve both as a scaffold for virtue and as a mask for vice. They can help support individuals to be compassionate, conscientious and trustworthy, but they can also help foster the belief that people have these good qualities even where these qualities are more or less absent in important respects.

The Shipman case, especially in the way it has been carefully and subtly analysed by Brian Hurwitz,[1] is particularly instructive in this regard. Harold Shipman's motives for killing his victims remain obscure and contested. (Indeed, he is used in Craig Webber's textbook on *Psychology and Crime*[2] as a clear example of someone who falls outside the typical motivational typologies of serial killers.) Although there has been much speculation about his psychological make-up, no consensus has emerged to explain his behaviour. The fact that it cannot be easily explained also means that it cannot easily be 'explained away'. On the surface, at least, Shipman seemed to fit the mould of the good doctor. It is this superficial similarity to the norm that is both disturbing and revealing. It is disturbing because it would be more comfortable for us to be able to point to something conspicuously 'strange' about Shipman that marked him out from the rest of us. (It should be said that with both Allitt and Shipman there were significant behavioural incidents in their earlier lives that could have caused suspicion but, in practice, these were not sufficient to prevent them from practising.) But it is also, for closely allied reasons, revealing – because Shipman is almost a paradigm example of the 'masking' worry that we have raised. As Hurwitz has shown, albeit expressed here in a rather cruder fashion, it was because Shipman so completely filled the role of 'good doctor' that he was able to do the things he did. He was not a killer disguised as a doctor; he was a doctor who, in addition to conducting a conventional practice, killed people.

Clearly, the kinds of harms that might be caused, or wrongs that might be done, by most people occupying professional roles are very different to these terrible crimes. As noted above, in many instances these might simply involve an element of what is treated legally as 'negligence' – the absence of the kind of care and treatment that should be expected; or even just a degree of what might be called 'moral negligence' – sometimes falling short in practice of aspirations and standards that individual professionals hold dear in principle. But it is important to be clear that: (a) occupying a professional role, in itself, does not and cannot serve as an 'ethical panacea'; and (b) putting people in professional roles carries risks (and not only advantages) for society. Whether for good or ill, there is something socially powerful about professional roles, a point we develop further in the next section.

Idealistic and critical readings of professionalism

The discussion thus far – partly by drawing upon some extreme examples – has indicated the potential for good and for harm that can flow from people occupying and exercising professional roles. It has, therefore, enabled us to begin to discuss one of the biggest themes in the study of professionalism – the contrasts between idealistic and critical readings of professions.[3] However, it should be stressed immediately that critical readings of professions do not principally depend on the fact that individual professionals can do 'bad things' – major or minor – but, more fundamentally, rest on the idea that there is something inherently troublesome about the generation of professional status and power. The core tension between idealistic and critical readings is whether professions and professionals exist to serve society, or whether they are in important respects harmful to society – whether, indeed, the 'image' of service to society masks different ends and interests (either those of professions and professionals themselves, or those of other powerful forces or agents).

Idealistic and critical readings need to be understood together because they are essentially different perspectives on the same process, perspectives that emphasize different facets of that process. For example, the special status of professionals can be interpreted in more than one way. In the establishment of professional groups, some people are being developed and licensed to support or care for others, but at the same time they are 'separated off' from others and given some elevated social status. This is particularly obvious for traditional professions such as medicine and law, which are typically seen, at an individual level, as allowing people to achieve a comparatively high social status and, at a social level, to mark out the boundaries of relatively powerful social groups. These associations do not apply so straightforwardly to other health and social care professions, but the same broad processes of 'upward mobility' and 'exclusion' apply to them. That is, when someone becomes a social worker or a nurse, for example, they are obtaining a job and securing a place on an occupational ladder and, although they may not think at all in these terms, they are making themselves eligible for social opportunities and roles which may feel powerful to their clients, and which are closed to others. This is not to deny that there are some hugely important, real and perceived, status differences amongst different health and social care professions, which we will come to shortly.

To understand such processes, it is important to recognize that there is a potential gap between individual motivations and social effects. Professional identity can be seen both from the 'inside' and from the 'outside'. Individuals will have their reasons to enter, and to work, within a profession – they may have ambitions for themselves and/or to change things in the world, a sense of direction and purpose. Here, the idea of a 'vocation' – of being 'called' or having a 'mission', exemplified in the cases of Nightingale and Schweitzer – is often cited. Although the idea of a vocation sounds rather lofty and grand, and the term may feel outdated to many, something similar can still be a routine feature of the lives of professionals – a sense of being bound up with something much bigger than oneself and feeling one *has* to make a contribution and that doing so realizes an important part of one's identity. However, whatever the 'inside story', professions also need to be understood from the 'outside'. Individuals cannot just invent professional roles. Professions are defined socially and, in some respects, professionals are like actors playing their parts. Professionals have broad 'social scripts' to follow, scripts that are established by traditions and institutions. This makes it possible, and important, to ask sociological as well as philosophical, questions about professional roles and identities. This gap between inside and outside perspectives means that we can be concerned about some of the effects of professional roles without necessarily being suspicious about the motivations of individual professionals.

Looking at professional roles from the outside enables us to see things which are not always visible, or in focus, from the inside (and vice versa). It enables us to think about the wood and not just the trees, and this also applies to analyses of the social functions and effects of professions. An individual practitioner may focus on some specific set of tasks and goals, but it is important to see these in the context of the overall effects of professional work. Although these effects can be analysed in idealistic or positive terms – for example, suggesting that professions support individuals and groups and help social life to proceed effectively and smoothly – much work in the sociology of professions has emphasized the critical rather than the ideal readings of professional work. In particular, an outside – and critical – perspective helps us to understand the linkage between professions and various kinds of social power. Specifically, professional roles are powerful in the way they shape the identities and agendas both of practitioners themselves and of service users, in the way they reproduce and create various forms of social hierarchy such as those relating to gender, class or ethnicity, and in the way they bolster powerful social interests and create social distance between people.[4]

We have already illustrated how the occupation of a professional role gives an individual a licence to 'invade' other people's lives, providing both the opportunity to benefit them and a potential mask for causing harm. Processes of professional socialization mould individuals to varying degrees so as to enable them to adhere to role expectations and fit into the relevant professional communities and working contexts. These socializing processes encompass, for example, ways of relating, talking and carrying oneself, dress norms, and purposes, values and beliefs. Much of this is often captured by theorists citing Bourdieu's notion of habitus – that is, the habits of mind and embodied dispositions associated with certain social positions.[5] Of course, practitioners are not identikit versions of one another and there are some limits to this moulding process; but, on the other hand, there are limits to how far individuals can deviate from the normative expectations of a professional group and still qualify as belonging to that group.

This is one respect in which professions and professional roles are socially powerful – that is, through the way they define, not only the identities but also the social and ethical sensibility of professionals themselves. But, in addition, health and care professions are socially powerful because of the way they, or the systems in which they are embedded, help to define the identities and lives of the users of the services they provide. In large part, it is professionals who determine what counts as normal or abnormal for service users, what counts as a real need or a legitimate preference that merits a social response, and what counts as an appropriate and reasonable kind of intervention. This is a pervasive phenomenon, but one well-known example is the area of pregnancy and childbirth where the framing of the issues, the labels that are attached to things and hence the experiences that are available to women have increasingly been defined professionally. A mother who is contemplating a 'home birth' following a discussion of its 'comparative risks and benefits' is already enmeshed in professional categories. More materially speaking, the reality of her choice in this matter will be determined to a significant degree by the way in which professional services have been configured.

Seen from this kind of critical perspective, professions, including health and social care, and thereby individual practitioners, whatever else they are, are agents of social control. They colonize common sense, define the parameters of what is thinkable and sayable, powerfully shape people's lives and experiences, police them in various ways and, in varying degrees but inevitably, are caught up in processes of oppression or exploitation. This crudely worded charge is elaborated, qualified and debated in multiple variations by sociologists drawing on different theoretical perspectives. For example, scholars inspired by Foucault's work highlight the ways in which professional power is deeply infused in all of social life and how professional discourses construct what count as legitimate ways of thinking about experiences, care needs and preferences and thereby at the same time marginalize or 'other' identities and behaviours that escape or transgress professional orthodoxies.[6] The Foucauldian perspective can be seen as complementary to Marxist and feminist critiques of professions as not only reflecting key social hierarchies in wider society but also as helping to reproduce them.

The traditional professions were at one time made up of exclusively male and predominantly white and middle- or upper-class people. Although this has changed substantially, there are still strong correlations between membership of a higher status professional group and privileged social identities. In this chapter, we have used the examples of medicine and nursing; in the case of these two occupations, the social construction of roles is very evident. The different roles are strongly 'gendered': the traditionally male role emphasizes 'cure' (associated with a technological attitude of applying science to get results); the traditionally female role emphasizes 'care' (associated with warmth, nurturing and the importance of relationships). The social role of doctors was historically analogous to the (now archaic) idea of head of household as compared to a more modest idea such as being a housewife; that is, the locus of power was unequivocally with the doctor, and the less powerful nurse role was constructed as essentially subservient to the 'male' role. Of course, again, things have changed in both domestic and working spheres, and boundaries and hierarchies have been eroded; but it would be foolish to imagine they have disappeared, or to fail to see the ways in which broader social and historical processes – whether relating to gender or other factors – continue to shape patterns in the division of labour and power. This is evident from the pervasive gender hierarchies across the professions, for example, with much greater proportions of men being appointed to senior positions. So even where professions, such as medicine, become more gender-balanced overall, not only do women remain less well represented at the top of the profession, but also the hierarchy of sub-specialisms is itself persistently gendered.[7]

On the basis of these brief remarks about both the social production and the social effects of professions, it is clear that even those who are concerned about the power of professionals will need to make some distinctions between the degrees and kinds of power exercised over service users by different professional groups. Once again, this is evident in the contrasting examples of medicine and nursing. Even though, as we have acknowledged (and as we will see further in the next chapter), the traditional stereotypes are no longer a perfect fit, the relative power and social status of doctors and nurses is different and – a closely related but distinct point – so is the average 'feel' of professional–patient relationships corresponding to these two sets of roles.

Membership of a professional group creates a degree of social distance between practitioner and service user. This is one of the ways in which the power of professionals is manifest to, and felt by, service users. Although there are many overlaps and exceptions, and although roles evolve, the general feel of some professional roles is more 'distant' than others. This question of social distance is a key one for all professionals in health and social care. Typically, such professionals have to work with individual clients on the one hand and institutions on the other. This can entail being empathetic and responsive enough to help or even 'befriend' a client, but it also means maintaining a certain professional distance, if only in order to retain objectivity and impartiality. Professionals can be more or less close to clients, but at the same time they do not operate solely in the sphere of the client; they are simultaneously more or less close to the structures and imperatives of the health and social care systems. The nature of these balancing acts is different in different roles; but in all cases relationships are inflected by professional power. As indicated above, such critical readings are not accusations about the motives of individual professionals. It is possible, and can be consistent, to maintain that the members of a professional group are operating in wholly well-intentioned ways and, at the same time, be concerned that their collective effects have important negative aspects which deserve critiquing.

Conclusion

In this opening chapter, we have sought to disrupt any assumption that professionals as individuals or professionalism as a set of occupational values are unproblematically or wholly good. With regard to individual professionals, we have tried to show how professional roles can provide both a scaffold for virtue and a mask for vice. With regard to the occupational values of professionalism, we have introduced the relevance of both idealistic and critical readings and, in particular, concerns about the widespread effects of professional power. Apart from indicating these complications and competing readings, we have deliberately skated around the idea of professionalism. We have not offered a definition or even a general account of what we mean by it. This is because the idea is a complex and contested one; as we will explain more fully in the next chapter, it would not only be difficult but also potentially misleading to provide a simple definition. In a sense, the whole of the book is our attempt at offering and exploring a general account of professionalism and the contests that are bound up with the idea.

In describing a practice or a set of activities as 'professional', people can be referring to a range of different things (over and above the idea that practitioners get paid or are non-amateur). First, they might just mean that the practice or activities are performed by someone occupying a certain kind of recognized social role (for example, a doctor not a road sweeper). Second, they might mean to highlight the fact that something is being done well – that it is an example of 'good practice'. In this very general sense, any kind of activity could be done 'professionally' providing it is done in accordance with the standards that apply to it (certainly road sweeping but also burglary and other crimes). Third, they might want to indicate that what is being done is not only being done well but that it is somehow an example of a particular kind of worthwhile activity and that the person doing it has some admirable and socially valued characteristics. This third sense can, therefore, be seen as a particular compound of the first two senses, combining specific kinds of activities with excellence of conduct within those activities. Doing medicine well, for example, would qualify but doing burglary well would not. It is in relation to this third sense that the idea of 'professionalism' is most often used. That is, it is most frequently used to allude to the admirable qualities and good practice of certain kinds of workers. We might commonly talk about a 'professional burglar', but it is less common, and somehow less fitting, to talk about the professionalism of a burglar.

Hence a discussion of professionalism leads us in these three directions. It requires us to think about the characteristics of that subset of jobs we classify as professions; about what it means to do a job well; and about whether there is something distinctive about doing work well within the subset of jobs that we label as professional. As we will go on to explore further, it is difficult to disentangle these threads. It is tempting to imagine that one of these threads is the crucial one for understanding professionalism and the other two could fall away into the background, but the more we try to make sense of the area, the more it is evident that these threads are entangled with one another. The account of professionalism that we offer in this book is based on the idea that understanding professionalism means paying attention to the nature of professional roles, to the ways in which these roles and associated standards are socially created, defined and legitimated, and to the qualities that are needed to occupy these roles responsibly, responsively and effectively.

CHAPTER TWO

Varieties of Professionalism

There is a danger that reference to the language of profession-alism has become so widespread as to be almost meaningless. In our routine conversations, we often use the term 'profes-sional' as a near-synonym for 'good'. For example, if we want to compliment our children for the way they have chopped the vegetables, we might say that they have done a 'professional job' – by which we mean a 'good job'; for example, perhaps they have cut them fairly evenly, tidily and willingly. In this usage the term clearly borrows its value from the more specific idea of a 'professional job' (the job a professional would do) but, of course, it does not mean exactly that because the vegeta-ble chopping of a professional cook or chef is a different thing altogether. Rather, it just borrows some of the connotations of the specific use – the notion that something is done (relatively) expertly and with care.

But the exploitation of the connotations of professional-ism also occurs in much more diffuse ways and on a much larger scale. The term 'professional' is increasingly used as a 'brand' to suggest that something or other is of good quality, admirable or desirable in some way. A web search of images for 'professional' indicates this. Amongst a wide variety of things thrown up are: images of good-looking, and apparently good-natured, men and women in smart suits, and suppliers of smart suits ('professional dress'); sleek, carefully designed and well-equipped hair and beauty salons; a selection of 'pro-fessional nail designs'; adverts for computers and computer systems, for exclusive social networking groups, and for train-ing in leadership and effective working. The list could go on.

An indefinitely large variety of occupations are encompassed, including professional carpet and upholstery cleaning, sound recording and mastering, and wrestling. Even if we take a supposedly archetypical 'non-professional' role such as 'road sweeping', it is not difficult to find organizations offering 'professional road sweeping' services. Furthermore, virtually any commodity on the market can come, and frequently does come, with the word 'professional' in their model name. There are professional drills and ladders, professional toothbrushes and toothpaste, professional exfoliating cleansers, professional telescopes and even – strange as it may seem – professional tea and coffee mugs. Here the implication is that these are versions that are, or are like, the ones used, or recommended by, people who are professionals, specialists or experts in some relevant sense.

These vague notions are not therefore completely meaningless. Rather, they symbolize a diverse set of connotations, images, associations and feelings. Looking at these examples and others, it is clear that there is a range of more or less closely linked tropes that are conveyed by these generic uses of 'brand professional'. It can be used to represent people who are good at things, have expertise and therefore can be trusted. Such people care about doing what they do. They thus have a host of potentially good qualities. They are thorough, committed, reliable and, depending on context, a whole galaxy of other things – discreet, tactful, approachable, kind, hard-headed, unrelenting and so on. The brand can be used to indicate activities and things that are not only high quality but also high status – respectable, smart, exclusive or elite. It can, in addition, be used to suggest that some environment or object is amongst the best available – beautifully designed and crafted, and consequently both aesthetically satisfying and high-powered, high-definition, high-tech and so forth. These different tropes and the emphases within and across them can be combined indefinitely into many cocktails of meaning. In other words, they provide a powerful well of resources for marketing, public relations, and endorsement in general in both formal and informal contexts.

How then are we to make sense of the ideas of being professional or being a professional in a world where these ideas seem to be applicable to almost anything and everything? If these ideas can be stretched into so many shapes and used for so many different purposes, is it sensible to ask, or is there any point in worrying about, what they actually, or should, mean? One way forward is to follow through the suggestion mentioned above in relation to the two senses of a 'professional job'; that is, the notion that there are secondary, peripheral or metaphorical uses of these ideas that 'borrow' some of the associations of a much more restricted set of primary or 'core' uses. This route would, for example, encourage us to think about paradigm cases of a 'professional job' and 'professionalism' and to see other uses as more or less pale reflections or more or less plausible extensions of these paradigm cases.

This line of enquiry might be seen as asking for the 'essence' of professionalism – an essence that makes up a relatively concentrated or diluted constituent of different cases. Some people, particularly those with certain kinds of practical or technical temperament, would be inclined to ask for a definition at this point: 'Just give me definitions and I will be able to apply the terms accordingly!' In what follows in this chapter and in the remainder of the book, we will respond to this challenge of finding some order in the apparent chaos of possibilities. We are broadly inclined to the view that the core–periphery picture is a useful one and in the next section we will begin to look for a 'core' sense by focusing on the idea of professions and what makes something a profession. However, we also want to stress the problems with sketching in the details of this picture, except in rather broad-brush ways. Similarly, whilst we do hope to convey something of the scope and boundaries of professionalism, we will not be offering a firm definition of it.

Our rationale for wanting to retain some of the open-endedness in play here is a positive one; that is, we would argue that, within limits, a fuzzier account is a more valid one, and that to offer firm clear-cut definitions in this area would, in important respects, be misleading and mistaken. This is because 'professionalism' is an example of what has been called an 'essentially contested concept'.[1] That is, in order properly to understand professionalism, it is vital to understand that there are disputes or contests about what it means. In this respect, it is like other important social concepts such as 'equality', 'freedom' or 'democracy'. In all these cases, there are different and competing conceptions of what these ideas mean. The contests between different conceptions of essentially contested concepts reflect the fact that they can be understood from within alternative political and ethical perspectives and in ways that are shaped by history and ideology. (This is why it is possible for idealistic and critical readings of professions and professionalism to exist alongside one another, as discussed in chapter 1.) To provide a rigid definition risks just asserting one perspective over others, thereby obscuring the contests that are built into the idea. It would be like defining social equality only as 'same treatment' *or* 'equal opportunity' *or* 'equal outcomes', and failing to see that these (and other) different competing elements are all bound up in the idea of equality. Our account of professionalism will, therefore, aim for a degree of closure and coherence whilst attempting to acknowledge and address the very substantial disputes surrounding this family of terms.

In the rest of the chapter, we will further unpack and explore the notions of profession and professionalism. Because the concept of professionalism is particularly difficult to pin down, we will begin by investigating it indirectly by focusing on the idea of a profession. Having reviewed some of the key sociological perspectives on the contested and historically emergent nature of professions, we will return to the idea of professionalism and summarize the distinctive nature of contemporary professionalism in health and social care under conditions of 'new professionalism'.

Professions

One place to begin thinking about the meaning of 'professional work' and professionalism is with the more concrete-seeming and circumscribed notion of 'a profession'. Which kinds of occupations do or should count as professions and which do not, and how, if at all, can we draw the lines here? As already indicated, this might provide important clues as to some of the connotations of professionalism. This is not a straightforward matter, as also indicated above, for example, with the reference to 'professional road sweeping'. Nonetheless, in everyday social life (and in categorizations used in social analysis) distinctions are routinely made between occupations that are 'professions' and those that are not. Paradigm examples of professions are high-status occupations such as medicine and law; paradigm examples of 'non-professions' are low-status occupations such as road sweeping or dish washing. (The fact that you can aspire to do these things, or indeed any job, 'in a professional way' does not seem enough to qualify the occupations as professions.) In between these two poles, there are of course many less clear-cut cases – including for example, teaching, occupational therapy or marketing – where some would resist using the label of 'profession' and others would insist that it is fitting.

One well-established approach to this demarcation issue is based upon 'trait theories' of professions; that is, upon identifying the 'traits' that give some occupations the status of professions. This is, indeed, one attempt to identify something like a core sense of profession and of professional work. The underlying assumption is that those occupations which are professions have some essential qualities in common. Once we identify the list of essential qualities or traits, we can then decide whether specific occupations qualify for the label, or at least where they are on the spectrum between undoubted professions and 'non-professions'. It is possible to find multiple such lists (of various lengths) in the literature but these tend to have a number of elements in common including, for example, the idea that professions require a considerable degree of specialist preparatory education.

A useful overview of the range of traits typically identified is provided in the *Encyclopedia of Social Theory*:

> While differing in their specific emphasis, there has been a common focus on eight broadly conceived characteristics that distinguish professions: (1) knowledge based on theory and substantively complex techniques, (2) mastery of knowledge that requires a long period of university based training that socializes trainees into the culture and symbols of the profession, (3) tasks that speak to relevant and key social values that are inherently valuable to societies, (4) practitioners that are oriented towards clients' welfare and service to the profession, (5) task performance characterized by a high degree of autonomy, (6) practitioners that exhibit long-term commitment to their work, (7) practitioners who enjoy a well-developed sense of community, and (8) a well-developed code of ethics that guides practitioner behaviour and defines the profession's core values.[2]

An alternative shorter but more consolidated list is provided by Daryl Koehn as part of her exploration of the distinctiveness of professional ethics:

> Professionals: (1) are licensed by the state to perform a certain act; (2) belong to an organization of similarly enfranchised agents who promulgate standards and/or ideals of behavior and who discipline one another for breaching these standards; (3) possess so-called 'esoteric' knowledge or skills not shared by other members of the community; (4) exercise autonomy over their work, work which is not well understood by the larger community; and (5) publicly pledge themselves to render assistance to those in need and as a consequence have special responsibilities or duties not incumbent upon others.[3]

It is possible to draw some provisional conclusions, and to raise some further questions, even on the basis of these two examples. First, certain key elements seem central – in particular, specialist knowledge, autonomy, social recognition and value, and service and ethical conduct. Second, it is clear that these traits do not neatly 'clear up' the question of which occupations count as professions. Whilst they seem to apply to a few 'classic professions' (although, as we will see, even this can be questioned), for most candidate occupations some traits apply more fully or uncontroversially than others. Third, such lists can be organized around slightly different axes. The first (typical) list centres on the characteristics of professional practitioners (ideas about professional groups and their social recognition are in the background); the second list explicitly highlights the social recognition of professions and the social function of professional organizations and roles. This difference of emphasis raises questions, which we briefly touched upon at the end of chapter 1, about the relationship between the characteristics of professionals and the characteristics of professions. The first list is effectively a summary of the special or desirable qualities of certain kinds of workers. The second list brings out the distinctive social role of professions and emphasizes the separation of, and distances between, members of professional groups and others. These largely positive accounts of professional roles and professional work and the distinctive and crucially important contribution that they make to the effective functioning of society were theoretically anticipated and elaborated in the 'functionalist' sociology of Talcott Parsons,[4] and before that by Durkheim,[5] one of the 'founding fathers' of sociology and a key influence on Parsons.

Trait theories were popular up until the 1970s and remain influential when people come to think about the nature of professions. However, since the 1970s trait theories – as typified by the first kind of list – have been subjected to much criticism for presenting the essential qualities of professional practice as essentially and simply 'good', and for neglecting the social power of professions. In other words, they largely reflect what we described in chapter I as the internal, idealistic and 'vocational' understanding of professional practice – the way practitioners might like to represent their role and work to themselves; but they can thereby obscure the more external and often critical understandings of professions which recognize the power of professions along with other related social advantages (status, income, etc.) of, at least some, professions. According to these critical perspectives, typical trait accounts disguise this bigger picture and merely reproduce an ideologically self-serving self-image for professionals.

Trait theories, whilst they have not disappeared, are now seen as rather old-fashioned. Since their heyday, accounts of professions have tended to evolve in two broadly complementary directions: (1) by acknowledging the intrinsic relationship between professions and social power; and (2) by emphasizing the diversity of professions and the contrasts between different kinds of professions. Both these shifts are prefigured in Johnson's Marxist-inspired analysis[6] and Larson's account of the rise of professionalism, arising out of a broadly interactionist sociological tradition.[7]

Johnson reacted to trait theory by questioning any assumption that professions were of a uniform nature and that they served everyone's interests and purposes equally. Rather, his analysis focused on the different historical forms through which professional groups gained their social recognition and power, based on a conceptualization of professionalism as 'a historically specific process which some occupations have undergone at a particular time, rather than a process which certain occupations may always be expected to undergo because of their own "essential qualities"'.[8] According to Johnson, professions can be loosely classified by the different ways in which social control over areas of work is maintained and exercised. In particular, he distinguishes between three kinds of professional power structures – 'collegiate' (e.g. medicine and law), in which members of the profession largely control themselves and their relations to the wider society; 'patronage' (e.g. accountancy and architecture), in which power is exercised as a result of negotiations between professionals and those who contract and pay for their services; and 'mediated' (e.g. social workers and nurses), where occupational control is not exercised directly by members of the professional group but by some other agency (most commonly the state itself) that sets the terms as to what and how professional work is to be organized and provided and whose interests are the ones to be served. Groups of professionals may be responsible for organizing their work on a day-to-day basis, and they may have a say over which purposes and practices they emphasize, but they do so within parameters set by, or negotiated with, the state or other mediating body. Professions vary, therefore, in their scope for both the collective autonomy of their professional groups and the individual autonomy of practitioners.

Larson's analysis contains some analogous points and differentiations. She considers the processes through which occupations become, or seek to become, professions and unpacks the social significance of these processes. Professionalization, she writes, is 'an attempt to translate one order of scarce resources – special knowledge and skills – into another – social and economic rewards'.[9] Her account distinguishes between, but highlights, the 'inseparability' of the two sets of social advantages arising from professionalization: market and economic advantages; and educational and status advantages. Larson notes that these two sets of advantages are often in tension with one another – that is, that the drive towards social status and respectability does not always sit comfortably with markets and the pursuit of money. On the other hand, she illustrates the important place of the 'ideological supports' provided by claims about respectability (for example, claims about gentility, disinterestedness or caring) in helping to secure professional status and to legitimize the resultant status inequalities between professionals and non-professionals (and between different professional groups). How far an occupational group succeeds in professionalizing will, on this account, depend upon their ability to convert their theoretical knowledge or practical skills into some combination of economic and social status. The kind of professional group they become will depend upon the kinds, and mixtures, of economic and social positions they manage to achieve. The sorts of differentiations between *types* of professions made by theorists such as Johnson and Larson provide a richer alternative to the idea that has sometimes been deployed that occupational groups can be classified according to their *degree* of professional status, for example, that occupations such as nursing or teaching might be classified as 'semi-professions'.[10]

Is social work a profession?

In 1915, celebrated US educationalist Abraham Flexner gave a lecture entitled 'Is Social Work a Profession?'[11] His conclusion was essentially a negative one, although he made his case tentatively and in a way that welcomed disagreement. Inherent in his argument is a kind of early trait account of professions based upon what he calls the 'unmistakable professions' of medicine, law and the Church. It is worth briefly revisiting his account and reflecting on some of the changes of the past hundred years, changes that mean that it is now much less contentious to argue that social work is a profession. Flexner sees 'intellectuality' as the first mark of a profession. A professional is not someone doing something purely manual or narrowly technical, but someone exercising their intellect and discretion in a way that involves taking both responsibility and risks. In order for professions to have this intellectual character, it is necessary that they employ knowledge that is not generally accessible; that is, it involves some specialist learning. The purposes of a profession need to be relatively well defined such that professionals 'operate within definite fields and strive towards objects capable of clear, unambiguous, and concrete formulation'. Finally, he suggests, membership of a profession is likely to be fully absorbing, and, as professions develop, they are increasingly likely to be devoted to 'well-doing' and advancing 'the common social interest'. Flexner compares various occupations (plumbing, banking and nursing) against this rough template and judges that they each fall short for one reason or another. His slightly more extended discussion of social work comes to the same, albeit heavily qualified, conclusion. In brief, Flexner takes the line that social work does rest upon intellectual elements and draws upon a range of specialist learning that extends beyond common sense. He also accepts that it certainly meets the criterion of being devoted to the common social interest. Nonetheless, he questions social work's professional status on the basis that the social worker is not an agent with the same level of responsibility and risk-taking that he attributes to the paradigm professions, but that social work is rather a supplementary profession that operates as a kind of 'mediating agency'. The idea here is that social workers do not take the ultimate responsibility for the well-being of their clients but depend upon referring them to individuals in other professions or services. In this respect, he sees social work as somewhat akin to nursing in that it embodies a kind of secondary agency; that is, one that ultimately refers back to the agency of the doctor.

This summary shows how trait theories have been used historically, but it also shows their limitations. Since Flexner gave his lecture, social work has obviously changed, but so also has the way we tend to think about professions. For example, what Flexner notes as the relative dearth of specialist faculty members and specialized publications in social work is something that clearly no longer applies. In addition, there is now widespread acceptance of more equal relationships and teamwork between members of occupational groups in education and social care in a way that makes the idea of purely secondary or borrowed agency seem largely out of date; and there can be no question that these days social work practitioners have to exercise higher levels of individual responsibility for cases and take risks based on their specialized understanding and experience. Furthermore, there have been very many changes in economic, social and political life since Johnson and Larson were writing, along with corresponding changes to structures of professionalism. For example, Johnson's distinction between 'state-mediated' professions, such as nursing and social work, and independent collegiate professions, such as medicine, has become a far less clear-cut one.

As Johnson and Larson and many other theorists since have highlighted (and, incidentally, as Flexner anticipates), conceptions of professions have also shifted over the past hundred years. In particular, less weight is now attached to the idea of the 'essence' of the profession. Rather, the emergence of the professions is now considered to be a historical process resulting in different kinds of professions with different forms of organization and different degrees of power and status. Once this diversity is recognized, the key issue is not to decide whether social work (or some other occupation) qualifies as a profession because it shares key characteristics with medicine (or some other paradigm), but to ask what is meant by, and what makes possible, different claims to professional status. We will not pursue this theme further here. However, in brief our view is that social work has a perfectly good claim to professional status, but, as we will discuss in the next chapter and later in the book, this claim can be undermined if the necessary social conditions are not in place to support social work professionalism.

The very many positive attributes associated with 'brand professional' with which we began can now be seen to reflect key elements in the professionalization projects undertaken by occupational groups – especially claims concerning specific expertise, quality and respectability. To achieve professional status, occupational groups need to demonstrate the social importance of their distinctive knowledge base and to put in place mechanisms (e.g. professional bodies, entry

standards, codes of ethics) to establish a recognized and pro-
tected social role and associated technical and ethical quality
standards. Professionals are practitioners who occupy these
roles and embody these standards, and professionalism is
the successful occupation and fulfilment of these roles and
standards. By extension, anything else described by the label
'professional' borrows these positive connotations. However,
it is clear that not all claims about professional status or professionalism amount to exactly the same thing. There are a
range of dimensions to professions (as indicated in trait theories) that might be more or less present in different cases
and which can be embodied in different forms and degrees of
professional organization and control, and there are different
personal qualities associated with professionalism and different perspectives on these organizational forms and personal
qualities – including both idealistic and critical perspectives.
There are also (to some degree shifting) 'pecking orders'
between professional groups according to the level of collective power and sanctioned social authority they exercise over
specific domains, with some professions sometimes seen as
relatively 'supplementary' to others, to borrow Flexner's idea;
and professional groups do not only maintain their boundaries with non-professionals but also defend their boundaries
with the other professional groups who operate 'on their turf'.
Finally – as we have tried to indicate – notions of professions
and professionalism evolve historically and are shaped by
broader social changes (discussed next and further in the
following chapter).

'New professionalism'

In recent years, there has been much discussion of new
forms of professionalism. The language of 'new professionalism' indicates, and on occasions is designed to promote,
a significant shift away from traditional conceptions of professionalism. There are a range of different changes that are

indicated by the language of newness but for ease of presentation we will highlight two facets here, both of which can be seen as a response to the social power of professionals – a 'rebalancing' of power between professionals and their clients; and a 'rebalancing' of power between organizations and managers, on the one hand, and professionals, on the other. Each of these facets provides a different sense of new professionalism. In the first sense, new professionalism means something like partnership-working, and in the second sense it means something like managed professionalism (or what we discuss below as organizational professionalism). Other developments in models of professionalism can, in many cases, be approached through the lens of the two shifts we are focusing upon. Notably, the rise in team-working, and inter-professionalism more generally, can be seen as a manifestation both of partnership-working (in an extended sense) and of managed professionalism. We will discuss these different versions in turn even though they coexist and in some respects can be understood as facets of some broader processes (these linkages are discussed further at the end of chapter 3).

New professionalism as partnership-working
In recent years, influential conceptions of professionalism in health and social care have been framed around ideas such as 'partnership-working' or 'person-centredness', partly to stress the need to close the power and status gap between professionals and patients or clients, and partly to re-stress the traditional notion that the goal of professional work is to serve the needs and address the concerns of service users. These kinds of shifts in emphasis pervade the policy and research literatures across the public service professions. Calls for a 'new', person-centred professionalism are, for example, as well established within medicine as they are within nursing. In the United Kingdom, a Royal College of Physicians report calling for 'new professionalism' stresses the values of 'well-being, dignity, partnership and mutual respect' and contrasts these with the old notions

of 'mastery, autonomy, privilege, and self-regulation', arguing, for example, that mastery 'can suggest control, authority, power and superiority – ideals that are not compatible with our view of the patient–doctor partnership'.[12,13] Very similar shifts have been recognized and called for in other national contexts. For example, a discussion of 'The Medical Workforce of the Future' in *The Medical Journal of Australia* stresses that 'Doctors will not be the all-authoritative figures' but rather 'they will need to understand team care' including 'patient engagement in decision making'.[14]

These new ways of constructing professionalism seem to have the potential to refresh thinking and practice in health and social care. They point in the direction of new kinds of relationships, often referred to as 'more equal' relationships. These new constructions maintain the key components of traditional conceptions of professionalism – the focus on the use of expertise and the maintenance of high technical and ethical standards – but they suggest a rather different interpretation of these things. A good illustration, and symbol, of these shifts is the gradual change of language in the area of medicines prescribing from 'compliance' to 'adherence' or even 'concordance'.

The language of 'compliance' refers to the patient 'following the doctor's orders'. The underlying assumption is that the prescriber has the biomedical and pharmacological expertise needed to identify the best treatment for the patient. This does not mean ignoring the patient. On the contrary, the prescriber must attend very closely to the patient, including the patient's account of their experience, if they are to come up with a correct diagnosis and an informed prescription. They must also have the skills to communicate their conclusions and their advice effectively to the patient. As well as striving to get the technical judgements right, they have ethical duties to explain the possible effects of the treatment, including possible side effects or uncertainties. This captures the basics of traditional professionalism in this area. Increasingly, however, it is thought that this way of thinking about prescribing is not enough, that something 'more', or different, is required by the new professionalism. In a nutshell, this refers to the greater involvement of patients both in decisions, within consultations, about the best choice of medicine and in the actual use of medicines following the consultation. This shift in emphasis has come about for many reasons. These include concerns about effectiveness (patients are more likely to use medicines effectively if they are involved) and concerns about ethics (patients deserve to be taken seriously and to have their own expertise respected). The terms 'adherence' and 'concordance', which are now generally preferred to the language of compliance, reflect different aspects of this shift in emphasis, the former capturing the idea of a patient actively following and 'owning' a course of action and the latter capturing the idea of a patient actively working in partnership with a professional to determine the best course of action. The language of 'concordance' is not used much outside of prescribing contexts, but the equivalent idea of 'shared decision-making' has become recognized as of central importance, and is much advocated and debated across healthcare contexts nationally and internationally.[15]

Of course, these changes in language are not necessarily fully reflected by changes in practice – this is one of many areas of healthcare reform where changes are much easier to imagine than to enact[16] – but they do usefully summarize (a version of) new conceptions of professionalism. In particular, what is clear is that notions of professional expertise and of high technical and ethical standards get reworked as we move away from compliance models towards concordance models. If patients (or service users more generally) are to be more involved in decisions, then professionals need the capability to enable, support and respond to this involvement. This is something more, and arguably much more demanding, than simply being able to clearly communicate the reasoning behind, and the potential benefits and risks of, their own recommendations. More specifically, the assessment of what counts as the technically 'correct prescription' alters. A correct decision will be one that reflects the relevant preferences of specific patients (for example, where there are choices to be made between comparable medicines or about matters such as the mode or frequency of adminis-tration) and not just the general preferences of prescribers about treatment regimes. Ideas about ethical standards shift in analogous ways. Treating a patient with respect, at least ideally, means treating their experiences, perceptions and preferences not just as relevant data for professional decision-making but as matters worth taking seriously in their own right including within decision-making partnerships.

New professionalism as organizational professionalism
New forms of relationships with service users represent only one way in which social change has influenced conceptions of professionalism. For example, new forms of governance have spread across society which in part take the kinds of tools and drivers that would once have been associated with the promo-tion of economic productivity and apply them to more diffuse areas of social life, including what might have previously been thought of as either the personal or public goods of health and social care. This involves a new emphasis on measuring work, target setting, the spread of budget consciousness and the values of efficiency and enterprise. In public services, for example, these changes have been manifest in the partly com-plementary, partly contrasting strategies of managerialization and marketization. These new forms of governance do not just represent external forces constraining work and professional identities, but they actually help to constitute new subjectivi-ties and identities. They are processes through which people begin to think of themselves and govern themselves in dif-ferent terms – for example, as responsible, self-disciplined and productive agents – sometimes discussed in Foucauldian terms under the heading of 'governmentality'.

   Julia Evetts has analysed the way in which the identities of professionals are increasingly shaped by the identities of the large-scale organizations that employ them.[17] This, she argues, has produced new forms of professionalism which are defined in terms of, and reproduce, organizational values. In practical terms, this means professional work and identity are increasingly shaped by bureaucratic norms, standardized procedures and output measures and by discourses of cost-effectiveness and organizational or departmental competitiveness. What Evetts calls organizational professionalism is a version of new professionalism which incorporates traditional, collegial conceptions of professionalism but reworks these older conceptions and inflects them to bring them into line with organizational logics.

We can return to the prescribing example to briefly illustrate this sense of new professionalism. Over recent decades, the prescribing of medicines in both hospitals and community contexts has been subjected to ever more advanced forms of surveillance and technological monitoring and modelling. At the same time, the growth of evidence-based medicine has supported the development of more closely defined and stricter national and local guidelines over prescribing judgements. These developments, in combination with institutional drug formularies planned with both effectiveness and cost in mind, have eroded, sometimes in subtle ways and sometimes bluntly, the traditional prescribing autonomy of clinicians. These days, for example, it would be impossible for a clinician to prescribe a very expensive drug when a cheaper option was available without at the very least their being mindful of the broader system and resource implications of so doing and in some cases having to seek special approval from some other agency or committee.[18]

As with partnership-working, this facet of new professionalism is rooted in constructive agendas. Just as it is, of course, typically considered a good thing that service users have a greater say both in the shape of the services they experience and in what happens to them individually, the 'evidence-based' movement, for example, stresses the importance of knowing 'what works' if you want to treat people responsibly. This may constrain autonomy in some respects but, it can be argued, 'What is the value of professional discretion if it is misdirected and provides worthless or possibly harmful treatments to people?' (This is not to deny that there can be dilemmas arising out of these constructive agendas; see chapter 5.)

Having used the same example to illustrate both facets of new professionalism allows us to see the ways in which contemporary practitioners have to renegotiate relationships in different directions. This includes their relationships with both service users and managers but within a much more extensive network of inter-professional and inter-institutional relationships. This in turn entails more toleration of professional 'boundary crossing' and more emphasis on equality of respect between professionals and not just between professionals and service users.[19] In the case of prescribing, professionals are being encouraged to enter into partnership with patients at the same time that they are expected to be mindful of system demands and constraints and to work in a coordinated way with colleagues, but this example could be generalized across the whole of the health and social care sector where similar patterns of change, norms and discourses circulate. The contemporary social worker, for example, is expected to be person-centred and to work in partnership with colleagues, clients and interested groups and at the same time is heavily regulated by organizational targets and standards. Professionalism, which is a complex series of balancing acts at the best of times, is peculiarly demanding under these circumstances.

Conclusion

The use of the term 'professional' to approve of things, or sell them to us, has become so widespread that it has become easy to lose sight of what, if anything, it is supposed to mean. In many of these instances, professional has seemingly become a near synonym for good. We have suggested that some progress can be made, in the task of uncovering a core range of meanings, by focusing on the idea of a profession. If we know what counts as a profession, and we see professionalism as picking out the positive qualities associated with professions, then perhaps we stand a chance of distinguishing between the 'root' sense of profession and professionalism and the very many extended or metaphorical senses. Up to a point, we would suggest, this is a helpful exercise. There are valuable accounts of the nature of professional roles that highlight both the social characteristics of professions and the personal characteristics of professionals. It seems sensible to see professionalism, first and foremost, as about the expression of these characteristics. Unfortunately, this does not take us as far as we might hope. This is because no definitive or fixed definition of a profession is available. First, there is contestation around what counts as a profession, with the boundary between professional and non-professional roles being a matter of dispute. Second, the nature of professions and the language of professions and professionalism are subject to historical and cultural variation. In the previous section, we highlighted just one aspect of this elasticity by briefly outlining the 'new' features of 'new professionalism' in health and social care. Nonetheless, the elasticity is perhaps only relative. If we keep in mind the possibility of some core sense of profession, whilst allowing for complications, then we may be able to construct a useful lens for understanding and advancing professionalism. We return to this challenge in chapter 4. Before then, however, we need to consider a fundamentally important worry – should we be assuming that the idea of professionalism still has relevance? An alternative might be to decide that professionalism, as it has been historically understood, is no longer that useful a category in a very different time, or even perhaps that it is impossible to realize anything recognizable as professionalism under contemporary conditions. This is the focus of the next chapter.

CHAPTER THREE

Impossible Dreams

In this chapter, we want to entertain the idea that professionalism has become impossible. We will take this idea seriously
and review a number of different reasons for thinking it is
worth taking seriously. Although this may seem rather a negative approach to the topic, we think it is actually a potentially
constructive one. The hope is that, by highlighting real-world
obstacles to professionalism, we will be left with a clearer
sense of the issues that those people – including us – who
are interested in supporting the professionalism of health and
social care workers need to address.

We will leave to one side worries that talk about professionalism is inherently bogus and assume that there could
be social environments and institutional working conditions
that make something worth labelling professionalism possible. But this leaves us with two sets of worries to consider.
First, as we have been indicating, constructions of professionalism evolve, and this suggests that many ideas people
have about professionalism may no longer have relevance
in a changing world. Second, and arguably a much more
important worry, is whether the relevant environments and
conditions to support meaningful forms of professionalism
are actually available for many (perhaps the vast majority of)
contemporary health and social care workers. For these workers professionalism may remain a theoretical possibility but
perhaps, once we 'stop and look', we will see that it is a practical impossibility.

In what follows, we will review some of the main reasons
for being sceptical about the possibility of professionalism

in the practical circumstances of contemporary health and social care. In the first part of the chapter, we will discuss social changes that seem to undermine the viability of conventional versions and associations of professionalism. These include challenges posed by the ever more complex division of labour, and by a reworking of the structural conditions that have traditionally been characterized as underpinning professionalism (according to trait theory, for example) – in particular, autonomy and collegiality. They also include a multiplication of different kinds and conceptions of knowledge and greater access to and ownership of knowledge by various publics. These changes resonate with a more general decline in deference and an increase in both democratic and consumerist currents in public life associated with the rise of 'lay' and social movements, on the one hand, and with free-market economics, on the other. All of this reinforces the need for us to collectively think about professionalism in new ways and helps to explain the emergence of versions of 'new professionalism' as introduced in the last chapter.

In the second part of the chapter, we focus more on the ways in which these broad structural changes combine with more specific changes to working conditions – such as intensified demands arising from financial constraints – in a way which appears to diminish, or even eliminate, the scope for anything worthy of the name professionalism, old or new.

This chapter may thus seem like a litany of negativity. We will be rehearsing and exploring one reason after another for being sceptical about talk of, or aspirations towards, professionalism. But, as we have noted, our intentions are to turn this into something constructive. We hope these themes will not only further illustrate the evolution of ideas relating to professions and professionalism but also directly and indirectly help illuminate: (a) how contemporary conceptions of professionalism need to be different from conventional conceptions if they are still to make sense and be viable; and (b) how demanding it is to exercise and underpin professionalism

in contemporary conditions. We will return to this constructive agenda in the conclusion and then stay with it for the
remainder of the book.

No more special occupations

An ever-growing group of occupations have called themselves
professions and have adopted the occupational value of professionalism. This is not necessarily something to be cynical
about but, given the important branding effects of such labels
discussed in the last chapter, we obviously cannot treat the
growth in 'professions' as capturing a simple fact about the
steady spread of professionalism. Indeed, we might be inclined
to ask, 'if nearly everyone is a professional, then does the idea
retain any significance?'

Traditionally, the idea of a profession referred to a rather
narrow set of occupations that were seen to have a particular societal importance and carried special status. Even at a
crude level, we might wonder if the meaning of the idea is
not somehow lost, or substantially diluted, if it is generalized very broadly. Imagine, for example, that everyone's job
title included the word 'president', or that everyone was given
an aristocratic title. This would not mean that everyone had
become special, but that a former kind of 'specialness' was
being dissolved. It may be that the notion of 'profession' is very
different from these other examples. It could be argued that
the issue of social status is not really that important in the case
of professions – not the crux of the matter – but a similar concern can be raised about the idea of some work having special
societal importance. The most restricted lists of professions
– for example, lawyers, clergy and doctors – have sometimes
been characterized as organized around a handful of fundamental 'goods' – justice, salvation or spiritual well-being and
health – which are of immeasurable importance to sometimes
vulnerable individuals who are, more or less, in need of various forms of representation, support and protection.[1]

In this picture, the status of these traditional professions is thus not about something superficial, like the snobbery that might attach to them, but reflects the special role of those who are in a position, and can be trusted, to provide and protect these foundational goods and act as champions of those who need them. This special status is a corollary of the importance we collectively attach to these goods. Although we hope not to be let down by getting shoddy goods from a retail assistant or a botched job from our local builder, these failures are not of ultimate importance. This restricted and traditional conception corresponds with a range of other notions that now seem rather 'old-fashioned'. The figures in these special roles were normally male, white and upper- or middle-class and they were often regarded as civic leaders or community elders who could help supply dignity and legitimacy to all manner of social proceedings. Their standing inversely reflected their small numbers. Of course, the privileged social position of these professional groups was also a product of other things. They were, in general, amongst the best educated members of the local communities in which they worked, and the social influence they exercised often went along with the opportunity to exercise and practise their professional discretion. That is, in the way they applied their expertise, and in their broader social contributions, they had a degree of autonomy which made a community leadership role possible for them.

The proliferation of professions changes this. It is partly a reflection of an increasingly complex division of labour in which we look in many different directions for specialist expertise – to nanotechnologists, arts administrators, software engineers, pilates teachers, graphic designers and so on. It is partly a reflection of a less hierarchical and deferential society, and one in which further and higher education have become open to many. In contemporary society, social authority is both more diffused and more contested. Health and well-being, for example, are still seen as of immense importance of course, but the authority of the 'local doctor', and even of the medical profession as a whole, is increasingly open to question and to challenge.

The decline of deference and 'client revolt'

There is no area in social life where authority hasn't been questioned. For example, people who are interested in arts and 'culture' are less likely to take it for granted that there is something distinctively valuable in traditional conceptions of high culture. More generally, although there remain various kinds of social pecking order, this has become complicated and contested. There is no longer, for instance, a widespread presumption that members of aristocratic families are one's 'social superiors'. Relationships between the generations are also 'flatter' than they once were, with the authority of parents and grandparents being continuously interrogated. Professional roles are not exempt from these changes.

An early and deservedly influential analysis of changes to professional–client relationships was Haug and Sussman's 1969 discussion of what they call the 'revolt of the client'.[2] Haug and Sussman reflect on US examples drawn from the 1960s (which is the decade that the start of many of the transitions summarized above is often attributed to), including hospital care, social work and university education, where the authority and relevant expertise of 'expert professionals' had been challenged. Amongst other things, their analysis illuminates the way in which professional expertise can be contested, especially when it strays into areas of social life where client groups or service users judge that they have their own firsthand and rich expertise, not least relating to their experiences and the conditions of their own lives. For example, they discuss individual and collective resistance by black people to prevailing social work and educational practices that do not reflect an understanding of black history, identity and exclusion.

More generally, Haug and Sussman's analysis reminds us that relationships between professionals and service users cannot be taken for granted. Relationships need to be built in the first place and then effectively sustained, and there are a number of ways in which these processes can fail or break down. Even when they are sustained, such relationships are not necessarily successful or satisfactory. So although their account focuses on revolt or organized resistance, lying behind this are other more or less visible and dramatic examples of relationship breakdown. Professionals may characterize certain individuals or groups as 'hard to reach'. Yet, from the perspective of these people, these same professionals and the services they provide might be seen as irrelevant, alienating or even hostile. Low uptake and high drop-out rates from services might, therefore, at least in some cases, be seen as silent testimony to the scepticism of people about the value and relevance of professional expertise. (Another well-known example of breakdown or 'disconnection' is the rise in litigation against professionals where individuals react to a sense of being let down or mistreated by entering into overt conflict with services.)

The decline in deference is bound up with other closely related and deep-seated social transformations. These include a much greater equality of access to information and sources of knowledge. This is partly produced by a closing of the gap between formal educational opportunities of professionals and many of their clients and partly by the extraordinary rise and penetration of information technologies which have levelled or at least reduced the walls that used to mark off specialist occupational or technical knowledges. This has created a climate in which any motivated individual can relatively easily find resources for research and self-education.

Indeed, all of this arguably needs to be seen in the context of a growing culture of individualization. As Pfadenhauer puts it, albeit in a rather sweeping fashion: 'the authority of professionals is thus being gradually hollowed out and undermined. Instead and increasingly, each individual is coming to demand that he or she, their interests and their system of values, be granted a special status and that an exception be made for them.'[3]

Nowadays, it might be said, everyone is special and everyone is a critic. In relation to professional roles, a high-profile version of this orientation is the 24-hour media scrutiny of 'scandals', 'crises' and 'poor performance'. Along with everyone else, health and social care professionals are the subject of both fair criticism and sensationalist scare stories. Under these conditions, the traditional postures of professional authority become less viable; rather, respect for one's role and expertise has to be continuously earned and negotiated.

An unsuitable world for vocations

Processes of social change impact fundamentally on social identities, including the possibilities of professional identity. One of the features associated with the traditional 'special' professions is that the identities of individual professionals were often very fundamentally bound up with their profession. As noted above, this was certainly true of their social identities – the local clergyman or family doctor was not only expected to contribute to the community, in role, in multiple ways, but it was also not easy for them to get out of their role, still less to be anonymous. And something analogous could be said about self-identity – on the traditional model, individuals invested a large part of their identity in their role. This is most conspicuous in the case of clergy where it is well understood by everyone that they devote their life to their calling. But, as we noted in chapter 1, the idea of having a 'vocation', and of dedicating oneself to one's role and work can make sense more broadly. It is possible to do certain jobs without putting one's heart and soul into it; one can imagine 'going through the motions' whilst one's thoughts and feelings were elsewhere and largely disengaged. But individuals with a vocation are not merely doing a job; they are arguably entering into a state of being.

There seems something rather old-fashioned about the idea of a vocation nowadays and we would suggest this is not simply a question of fashion. There have been a host of social and cultural changes that mean the idea of a vocation is not easily combined with contemporary mores. There is so much more physical and geographical mobility which means individuals are not 'trapped' by the perceptions and expectations of the people immediately around them. There is increasing scepticism, and more toleration of a moral relativism, about people's underlying motives and values. This means that, even where individuals feel moved by profound beliefs and feelings and wish to act with moral seriousness, they are more likely to 'make light' of this fact or disguise it.

The considerable reflexivity about social and self-identity characteristic of modern societies creates a sense that people not only have complex and hybrid identities but also that they can, through choice, regularly re-invent themselves. Indeed, it is possible to argue that the project of identity building – as manifest, for example, in the CV – has become the most recognized, and perhaps central, way in which people orientate to 'careers' these days, rather than, one might worry, through a dedication to the substance of the work. Seen perhaps over-cynically, this looks like a shift from a focus on committing to and investing in one's work to a focus on investing in oneself. Against this background, it is not surprising to find Hafferty and Castellani, writing in the context of the United States but with unquestionable international relevance, talking about new versions of professionalism, including 'lifestyle professionalism' and 'entrepreneurial professionalism'.[4] In these versions of professionalism, the commitment to an occupational role is there partly because it serves other goods – a satisfactory work–life balance, or a platform for other activities including money-making – rather than as an end in itself. (Critics of the professions might, of course, want to insist that it has always been this way.)

None of this means that it is impossible to have a sense of

vocation in the contemporary workplace, but it does suggest that related commitments and identities are likely to feel less like a 'fact' both to others and to oneself, and that it would be understandable should practitioners choose to wear their vocation more lightly, self-critically or even with some sense of irony. This is one of the ways in which some of the traditional associations of professionalism can seem to be 'out of step' with the times.

In the chapter thus far, we have raised some questions about the relevance of conventional conceptions of professional roles, authority and identity to contemporary social life. The ground we have covered, therefore, also helps to explain why conceptions of professionalism have needed to evolve, resulting in the emergence of discourses around 'new professionalism'. In the remainder of the chapter, we question whether these new versions of professionalism (even if we assume they are coherent) are practicable in a changing workplace.

Working at the limit

Changing social conditions impact directly on the conditions of work in the health and social care sector. This is particularly obvious when we come to think of professions as a 'mass' rather than an 'elite' phenomenon. In an era of 'mass professionalism', the social context and organizational underpinning of much work labelled as professional does not support the working conditions conventionally associated with professions.

In the public sector in particular, health and social care practitioners work under considerable pressure. We have seen a long period of rising demand for health and social care at the same time that public expenditure has been under control. The continual refrain of policy makers has been that we need to 'get more for less', with services expected either to implement cuts or to find 'efficiency savings' so as to contain the rise in costs. This has meant that reinvestment in infrastructure is often slow and patchy and that practitioners' workloads have tended to intensify – that is, that individuals and teams are expected to deal with more patients or clients per day, sometimes with reduced resources. In some instances, service redesign (for example, improvement in the technologies that make day surgery possible) has enabled these efficiencies. In other instances, the result has been to make staffing levels precariously low – either because a few sickness absences can bring staffing levels below what is needed to provide even a minimal service or because the staff employed have to push themselves to the limits of their resilience to manage the necessary workload. These forms of intensification are, of course, not simply physically challenging – leading to tiredness or risks of injury – but they are a source of considerable stress to individuals who may feel that they cannot cope or feel that they do not have the psychological and emotional resources needed to look after themselves, support one another and – above all, of course – look after their clients as fully as they would like.

Human beings can be made to work more efficiently, just as engines or computers can, but there is a danger that, if this concept is pushed too far, the side effects will be quite serious. In a nutshell, what is at stake is not only a professional's own health but also their 'humanity' – their capacity to draw upon their full human resources of empathy, good humour and imagination. Under these circumstances, it is difficult to know what to make of the idea of professionalism. It is possible that practitioners may be complying with the minimum standards of good quality and safe provision but may be failing to 'give of themselves' in ways that they aspire to. It is, of course, also possible that they will constantly be at risk of falling below such minimum standards and that across a service, especially one with pockets of unsatisfactory infrastructure, tired equipment and low morale, enough individuals will cross this line to produce multiple examples of poor care and system failure. Even if someone were to question whether such risky working conditions are actually present in current health and social services, it would be irresponsible to deny that such conditions represent a hazard that needs consideration. The potential for good quality work does seem to depend upon drawing some limits to intensification and resource constraint and focusing on the humanity and well-being of staff as well as of those being cared for.[5]

Stuck in the middle

It is not only time and other resources that have been squeezed by the social context of contemporary public services. Professional autonomy has been squeezed too. Autonomy has long been taken to be a key feature of professions and professionalism and is usually prominent in trait theories. The assumption is that both individual and collective autonomy are important instrumental conditions for applying expertise because they allow for the application of expertise in diverse circumstances and cases through the use of experience-based professional judgement. Some people may also see them as a sign of, and intrinsic reward for, the special status of professionals as, in this respect at least, relatively privileged workers. To work as a professional is, in short, not to be told what to do and not to feel obliged to jump through hoops devised by others but to be able to steer one's own course by making one's own independent judgements under conditions defined in large measure by the collective power of one's professional organization. As we saw in the previous chapter, as more groups of workers became professionalized, they did so often with reduced expectations about levels of both individual and collective autonomy.[6]

So it is arguable that assumptions about the possession of professional autonomy apply less and less to most current health and care workers. Indeed, even if they did once apply to a subset of such workers – and doctors are the paradigm case – then the social changes we are reviewing suggest that they may no longer apply even to this minority, except in a considerably qualified way. In large part, this is because of the rise of the 'organizational' model of professionalism (introduced in chapter 2). All practitioners have become subject to ever stronger and more carefully elaborated forms of governance. These embody both visions of good practice and sometimes overlapping, sometimes competing managerial constraints and institutional expectations from their employing organizations. Similarly, the other aspect of 'new professionalism' – the widespread notion that practitioners should be more responsive to patients or clients – has implications for professional autonomy. The relative power of service users – whether construed as citizens involved in service planning or evaluation, as customers or 'quasi-customers' of services, or as 'partners' in provision – has risen in recent years and there is a prevailing orthodoxy that this is broadly a good thing and should be promoted more widely.

Similar points about changes to the autonomy of the individual practitioner can be made in relation to the rise of 'team-working' in health and social care. As with the other aspects of new professionalism, there is a credible and convincing rationale for the value of intra- and inter-professional teamwork. It makes sense to ask the individual practitioner to coordinate their activities with colleagues and thereby to 'pool' their autonomy so as to collectively provide a 'joined-up' service. Nonetheless, this does mean that some individuals – especially those with less power or status in a group – may be left feeling relatively 'unfree' to advance or pursue their own vision of what is best for a patient or client in order to comply with the prevailing practice of the group. At best, this situation does not look quite like the traditional picture of the individual practitioner independently sailing their solo professional ship but, in the case of more junior or less powerful practitioners, it may sometimes feel as if there is very little scope for any meaningful expressions of autonomy.

The result is that professionals can increasingly feel themselves to be squeezed from all sides: not only do they not 'call all the shots', but they can, in extreme cases, wonder whether they have any meaningful room for manoeuvre between the expectations and norms of managers and colleagues and the demands of users. This is not meant to imply that all such changes in the locus of influence are a bad thing. On the contrary, as noted in chapter 2, these changes are represented as – and many can reasonably be seen as – 'advances' in the quality of care. But these changes clearly raise the question of what kind of autonomy, and how much of it, practitioners can exercise in these new conditions.

Forms of 'new professionalism' – summarized above and in the previous chapter – have emerged as ways of adapting to the many social changes reviewed in this chapter, not least the need to balance the power and autonomy of professionals. But the issue arises as to the point at which levels of individual and collective autonomy become too low for meaningful forms of professionalism to still exist.

Standardizing the person?

This worry about loss of autonomy has been most strongly felt and expressed in relation to the powerful effects that managerial forms of governance have had on public services.[7] One way of summarizing such concerns is to see them as about the ways in which both practitioners and the people they are dealing with are being made to fit into narrow moulds – or are being 'standardized'. Services seeking 'efficiencies' and also wanting to secure the demonstrable accountability of practitioners have often prescribed quite specific outcome targets and modes of working, and underpinned these with performance management models, including systems of incentives orchestrated to bring practitioner priorities into line with institutional priorities. In some instances, these might be justified in terms of evidence-based rationales, but they are often underpinned by looser institutional contingencies, designed to contain costs and promote institutional consistency and cohesion through uniformity of training, provision and audit.

Under these circumstances, practitioners can feel as if they are being reduced to 'cogs in a machine' – that their jobs are being transformed into those of factory operatives who have formulaic roles with no discretion (and, in principle, could be replaced by robots). No doubt this characterization (and perhaps some of the feelings of frustration that get expressed in this context) are exaggerated; but the underlying worry is a real one that cannot be easily dismissed.

There are some very good arguments for standardization. Often variation in treatment is merely a sign that some people are getting bad treatment. If we have some idea of 'what works', the next question that naturally arises is how we can disseminate those practices that work across the system. But there is also a seeming paradox that the rise in defining, and 'system re-engineering' for, good practice has coincided with the rise in calls for person-centred care or 'personalization'. There is a considerable tension between the pressures within the system for standardization and the rationale for person-centredness. This applies both to those pressures that arise from institutional efficiency and those (overlapping sets) that stem from appeals to scientific research. The establishment of official norms and standard working practices, 'care pathways' and so on is based on generalizations. Sometimes generalizations may be an expression of some statistically significant piece of evidence. This is an advantage of the evidence-based practice model which tells us, for example, what interventions are, statistically speaking, more or less effective and it is therefore a useful heuristic for thinking about how to approach an individual.[8] Sometimes general rules are made to support the smooth running of institutions and to achieve efficient administration, deployment of staff, procurement of goods and services, and accounting systems. But generalizations do not always work for, or apply in a straightforward way to, individuals. And this is true both for individual service users and for individual practitioners.

Even evidence-based scientific generalizations – and this

is well understood by experienced practitioners – cannot be applied simply or directly to individuals. Individuals' problems will occur in the context of a range of other problems that need to be taken into consideration (for example, symptoms and diseases co-occur); there may be distinctive physical, psychological or social factors which mean individuals do not respond in line with statistical expectations; and – just as important – individuals may not value the typically desired outcome built into the study (that is, an individual may prefer no intervention or a generally less-approved intervention that has a balance of effects that suits them and their lives). The particularities and complexities of individuals are also not always served by what we might label 'bureaucratic generalizations'. Here too there can be very significant tensions between general principles and the needs and preferences of individuals. Of course, it is important not to be utopian about this. Not every possible variation between, or preference of, every individual can be fully responded to – the resource and organizational implications of this would be unrealistic. However, it is crucially important that practitioners have a significant degree of 'elbow room' to adapt their practices to individual cases, including, in some instances, to make exceptions to bureaucratic norms. Without this elbow room, they cannot meet the individuals in front of them as full persons and respond to their complexity as social and human beings, and – this also means – they are effectively not able to act as individual persons but merely as functionaries of a system. Whether or not these 'person-denying' characteristics exist within contemporary health and social care systems is disputed, but there is a plausible case for saying that it is a genuine threat to these systems and may already be a reality for some practitioners. In such cases, it seems that measures taken in large part to promote robust and cost-effective systems and to ensure that expertise is properly embedded in care practices – in short to underpin professionalism – risk undermining other facets of professionalism, such as those relating to individual discretion and individualized responsiveness. (We return to these worries about standardization and the question of what, if anything, can be done about them in chapter 6.)

Conclusion

Although we have rehearsed various reasons for concern about the very feasibility of professionalism, we have done so more in the spirit of realism than of pessimism. We are not inclined to the view that professionalism is an impossible dream. Indeed, for the remainder of the book we want to focus on the positive possibilities for professionalism, including the challenges of enacting and supporting it. The factors that we have considered develop and reinforce the message of chapter 2 that professionalism is historically shaped and is interpreted through evolving conceptions and models. Many contemporary professions never conformed to the self-governing forms of collegial professionalism that once formed the key archetype of professionalism, and traditional professions have themselves also, in many respects, moved away from this archetype. But this does not mean that practitioners cannot, in principle, exercise new forms of professionalism which retain some of the shape and resonances of the older forms. However – and this is a theme we have focused on particularly in the second half of the chapter – the 'in principle' possibility is only part of the issue. There are very important empirical questions to be asked about whether (and, more specifically, when, where and why) the social conditions for practising professionalism are – or are not – in place for large numbers of health and social care practitioners.

In the next chapter, we will begin to sketch a broad conception of professionalism – as the accomplished exercise of expertise-based social authority – that we believe is worth identifying and defending. This is a conception that we see as largely continuous with the models of professionalism reviewed in chapter 2 but which needs revisiting and

reinterpreting for contemporary social and working conditions. To prepare the ground, we think it is worth returning
to the analysis of Haug and Sussman from nearly fifty years
ago.[9] They see the growth of 'client' critique and resistance
as signalling necessary changes for notions of professional
expertise and authority. In particular, on their account, professionals were increasingly less welcome, and less legitimate,
when they attempted to extend their influence beyond the
immediate sphere of their specialism. The implication of this
would, they imagined, be that professional knowledge would
become defined in ever more circumscribed, technical and
'niche' ways. In other words, clients would look to professionals only to provide the specialist knowledge that the clients
lacked and could not obtain in some other way. Or, at least,
they would increasingly resist the notion that professionals
merited, and should exercise, some broader influence over
their lives.

This vision of the emerging role of the health and social
care professions might be understood by analogy with, for
example, independently minded individuals or groups who
are 'self-building' their new houses. By and large, they just get
on with it, using their 'amateur' expertise. But, from time to
time, they hit a snag about planning or execution that requires
them to turn to a specialist – a structural engineer, a lawyer,
an internet expert or some such. They do so, not looking for
general guidance about their plans, but only for very specific
pieces of the puzzle they are solving. By analogy, one might
imagine that we are all, individually and collectively, 'building' our own lives and we do not need, and may justifiably
resent, any implication that professional groups should do
more than provide the specific expertise we lack (including,
of course, any presumption that they should tell us directly or
indirectly how to live).

At the same time that they provide this vision of the possible
future of professional knowledge, Haug and Sussman provide
an extremely illuminating analysis of the response (already

manifest at the time of their writing) of professional groups to 'client revolt'. In particular, they focus upon the notion of 'co-option'. This is the business of professional groups forming links with lay individuals and social groups and thereby incorporating them into the sphere of influence of the professions, for example, by including them in the committees of professional organizations and, more broadly, in significant decision-making fora at institutional or micro-levels. This process of co-option breaks down the social distance between professionals and clients and, more specifically, gives some recognition and voice to lay individuals and groups, helping to legitimize their perspectives and the relevance of 'lay expertise'.[10] But, of course, it is also a response which can be seen as designed to bolster professional legitimacy and to dampen down active resistance towards it.

Looking back over half a century, it seems to us that these two elements of Haug and Sussman's analysis (specialization and co-option) are still highly relevant to understanding contemporary professionalism and, we would argue, it is possible to see them as much more closely related than was obvious then. A contemporary analyst would do well to think about professional expertise in the light of both these categories. The idea that professional groups, if they are to maintain a meaningful social role, need to define and occupy domains of specialist expertise, and that the boundaries of these domains are constantly in danger of erosion, remains salient. However, there have also been some developments in relation to conceptions of relevant expertise that can be connected to the idea of 'co-option' and the increasing imperative to work *with* communities and service users. Professional expertise, especially in health and social care, is not just specialist and technical but also includes 'relational expertise' (although the way these kinds of expertise are combined and balanced obviously varies according to role), and, if professionals are to retain legitimacy and, more importantly, to do something socially valuable, then both are needed.

There are strong resonances here with the two facets of 'new professionalism' that we summarized at the end of chapter 2. As we noted there, the two facets – organizational professionalism and partnership-working – can both be seen as about moderating the social power of professionals. They both represent a response to general social climates in which the legitimacy and radius of professional authority is less taken for granted and more subject to negotiation. They both represent currents of 'demystification' in relation to professional expertise – although with rather different emphases. Organizational professionalism partly rests upon and reinforces a concept of professional expertise as something that can be codified, measured and regulated. Partnership-working partly rests upon, and reinforces, the idea that expertise is more distributed across, and must include effective communication and 'bridge building' between, practitioners and service users. These two facets do not always fit together neatly and they can be combined with different emphases,[11] but, in broad terms, the drive behind these notions is to retain the relevance and potential of professionalism in a more sceptical and demanding world.

CHAPTER FOUR

Licensed to Care

How can we salvage the idea of professionalism from the 'wreckage' reviewed in the previous chapter? In this chapter, we will elaborate a broad positive conception of professionalism and defend its relevance and importance. The account we offer builds upon themes introduced earlier in the book and seeks to start pulling them together. Rather than exploring the range of possible versions of old or new professionalism, we want to outline a very general picture. In the following chapters, we will fill out this picture by exploring the challenges of underpinning and enacting professionalism in contemporary conditions. This chapter thus provides the fulcrum of the book.

We are interested in professionalism as an ideal in two closely related senses. First, we are interested in specifying an 'ideal type' – that is, an abstract conceptualization that attempts to capture the 'crux' of professionalism. Second, we are interested in getting at the way notions of professionalism connect with the 'ideals' of practice – practitioners' hopes and visions about the significance of their work, and service users' sense and appreciation of what they have felt and judged to be particularly valuable or 'best practice'. We should stress from the start that we do not see this positive picture as somehow cancelling out the concerns and problems associated with professionalism. This is a territory in which lofty aspirations and successes are necessarily entangled with human frailty and failures. But, we suggest, talking about ideals is compatible with acknowledging that many things are not ideal and that legitimate worries attach both to ideal types and to practice ideals.

We can use 'friendship' as an analogy here – both to explore the notion of an ideal type and to illuminate some of the ambiguities surrounding professionalism. We can imagine an ideal type of friendship – which, very roughly and in brief, might be something like 'a friend is someone who is interested in and cares about you and your well-being for your own sake and who shows this through their choices and actions, including the way they prioritize their time (and where these things are reciprocated)'. This captures something about the nature of friendship and the invaluable role it plays in our lives. Nonetheless, it is possible both to see the immense value of friendship and also ask sceptical questions about it both as an abstract ideal and in practice – is there not something inherently exclusive about friendship and does that not potentially cause problems? It may mean, for example, that friendship reproduces certain kinds of privilege – with the friends of privileged people ending up with a larger share of what is due to them on some other basis, not least need – or that patterns of friendship tend to sustain social distances between groups. Likewise, we may look at a particular act of friendship in practice and be moved by the generosity of spirit it manifests but still recognize that there are other elements present in the cocktail of dispositions and motivations lying behind the act – perhaps elements of insecurity, anxiety, 'trading' and so on. However, whilst recognizing these ambiguities and ambivalences – even seeing them starkly – we can still also see the presence, and the nobility and beauty, of the friendship act as a real-world expression of ideals. More generally, it is a crude mistake to see something – whether friendship or professionalism, for example – as *either* altruistic *or* self-centred. It is very common for there to be elements of both in individual and social action; furthermore, and even more importantly, these categories and this distinction arguably fail to get close to the heart of very many of the things we do quite routinely where we are moved to act for 'reasons of love' understood in the broadest sense.[1]

An example

Caitlin and Tomasz are very grateful to have Helen in their lives. Helen is the specialist cancer nurse who has been helping them look after their son Erik over the past two years. Their world has been turned upside down by Erik's illness and the emotional and practical load they have been facing exceeds anything they feel equipped to cope with. Helen has not been able to make things OK. Indeed, despite Erik's good humour and resilience, the situation has often felt unbearable. But Helen has somehow helped to make the experience of this unbearable load more manageable. Helen is a 'paediatric outreach oncology nurse specialist'.[2] She works with families and supports them at home and in their interactions with the health system. Caitlin and Tomasz value Helen for many interconnected reasons: (1) Helen understands the illness and the treatment – when they have been worried about the change in the chemotherapy regime, she has been able to discuss the clinical reasoning and clarify the details with them; (2) she is technically capable – hers were a very reassuring pair of hands when they thought the central line (through which Erik gets his treatment) was not functioning properly; (3) she is trusted, and listened to, by all of the other people who have come into their lives on a regular basis (including their GP, community nurses, teachers, social workers and hospital staff) – she has been able to help navigate a path through what would otherwise have been a bewildering scene and to make the right demands on, and have productive influence over, other practitioners; (4) she is just 'there' – Helen is at the end of phone when they need advice and she has often been there in person on scary days – sharing a cup of tea, and sometimes even sharing a laugh despite everything; (5) she is an experienced guide in an alien landscape. This is not just in terms of the working of the system, or the symptoms and treatment, but also in relation to their emotional landscape, including the continuous anxiety and fear that seems to have entered into their own bloodstreams. Whilst everything is new to them, the sense that it is a domain with which Helen is familiar is in itself somehow comforting.

Helen likes to be appreciated but is wary of being idealized by the families she supports. She loves her job, even though she finds it extremely demanding at times, and she knows she is not a saint. She aims to fulfil the role to the best of her ability, but there have been a few times when she has felt more disillusioned than dedicated. She has also made mistakes occasionally – luckily nothing too serious to date. For the most part the work feels very fulfilling and she finds that she cannot draw strict boundaries around it. It is not just that she has to be flexible about time, but she gets drawn into the families, sometimes quite significantly, and has found herself genuinely sharing the grief at those funerals she has chosen to go to. Luckily, she also has a stock of happier outcomes and positive memories to draw upon, and she gets good clinical supervision from a colleague who also regularly reminds her – although she doesn't need much reminding – of the importance of her non-work life and the need to maintain a balance. The work–life balance issue is important to her, partly because she wants to be able to continue in the work for several more years and she has seen many of her colleagues suffer 'burnout' quite quickly – an occupational threat she seeks to push far into the distance.

This quick sketch of one professional role – seen from the outside and from the inside – indicates the picture of professionalism we are hoping to paint more fully in the remainder of the chapter. It also, in a minimal way, conveys some of the dimensions of professional roles that may not be captured by abstract accounts. We are arguing that the nature and value of professionalism is found at the intersection of 'expertise' and 'social influence'. In health and social care, for example, some people – like Helen – have both the know-how and the social licence and legitimacy to care for others. Helen is 'a professional' in the sense that she is a member of a professional group with a particular social role, and she strives to be 'professional' in the sense of her performing her role conscientiously and to a high standard; and (as we suggested in chapter 1) in order to understand professionalism, we need to see the way these two things fit together. Helen has some socially recognized 'know-how' that enables her to make a contribution and gives her certain kinds of influence and 'powers' (for example, in moving in and out of hospital wards, communities and homes); and both the know-how itself, and its recognition, is bound up with technical and ethical standards. In short, Helen has *'expertise-based social authority'*.

According to this account, there are two key dimensions to professionalism, dimensions which can be considered separately but which only fully make sense when we focus on the ways in which they intersect: professionalism as a mode of social coordination; and professionalism as the embodiment of admirable characteristics, values or dispositions. We will say a little about each of these in turn and then try to unpack the implications of combining them more fully.

Professionalism as a mode of social coordination

Eliot Freidson has famously illuminated the first sense by analysing professionalism as a 'third logic', that is, as something separate from, and somehow complementary to, the ways in which social life is orchestrated by markets or by state-related bureaucracies.[3] Helen's role might be constrained and supported both by markets and by bureaucratic rules and procedures but it does not seem to be completely 'captured' by them. Markets organize social life by bringing together buyers and sellers in complex ways – people will, for example, have sold and bought the drugs and equipment that Helen uses. State bureaucracies are good systems for organizing and allocating services fairly – people will, for example, have planned the service Helen works for and made sure her job description is drawn up and her salary is paid on time and so on. These two modes of social coordination are certainly relevant here, but it seems that Helen's work as an individual professional, and the work of the broader specialist community of which she is a member, also embodies a form of social influence and social coordination that transcends these other two modes and can be seen as operating 'in addition' to them.

The paediatric oncology outreach service, and the work of individual professionals like Helen, deploys the (multi-faceted) expertise of specialist nurses to help make the world more responsive, or at least less indifferent, to the needs and purposes of people like Caitlin, Tomasz and Erik. This involves helping to shape and coordinate aspects of the social world, including local and micro-factors (such as arranging and practising effective and flexible telephone support) and national and macro-factors (such as revisions to hospital–community working relationships). It is arguable that the other two modes of coordination are ill-equipped to play this role. They seem likely to fail to 'see' and to 'act' in the required ways. The needs and preferences of the families are very specific, varied and context-sensitive; addressing them requires specialized understanding and skills. Families are under pressure and vulnerable; they are not in a good position to act as consumers; nor is there likely to be a marketplace sufficiently differentiated to be tailored to their demands in any case. Bureaucracies can be flexible but only in relatively broad-brush ways. They cannot realistically anticipate and plan for the specific needs and preferences of individual families or for the patterns of team-working that might operate best in different community and service contexts. There is a clear role here both for professional expertise and for professional influence in the form of specific instances of advocacy and more ongoing and structural service co-design functions.

We should stress that we are setting out an ideal type here, and our adoption of Freidson's notion of the third logic is part of that. In practice, the three logics cannot be neatly separated out, and nor is professionalism the only example of a third logic sitting between the state and the marketplace. As indicated in the discussion of organizational professionalism in chapter 2 (and Evetts' analysis drawn upon there), organizational logics have become increasingly hybrid, often inflecting professional norms with either bureaucratic or market forms of rationality (or both simultaneously). However, we would argue that, whilst these logics merge in real-life contexts, it is still possible to separate the idea of coordination through professional expertise from other forms of social coordination (indeed, this is what labelling merged forms as 'hybrid' depends upon). It would also be more accurate to talk about professionalism as *a* third logic because analogous stories might be told about other forms of social coordination that are not fully captured by the state or markets, including parts of the voluntary and charitable sector, civil society more generally or even self-organizing social or political movements. These other forms of third logic can be seen as variously complementary to, or rivalrous with, professionalism as a mode of social coordination. They too can also exist in hybrid combinations, as reflected, for example, in concerns about charities becoming more like businesses or voluntary work becoming more professionalized and so on. Whilst acknowledging these important complications, we will largely leave them aside here.

Professionalism as the embodiment of admirable qualities

Talking about 'expertise' can easily make it sound as if it refers to something dry or technical. In many people's minds, it conjures up the idea of academic knowledge and the factual contents of books and curricula. But, as is clear from the case of Helen, whilst expertise includes 'book learning', it ranges far more widely than that. Indeed, some of the relevant know-how can be about social and emotional matters, involving more than the intellect, drawing upon the whole person. Caring for the family in this case involves 'being' a certain way and, within limits, 'giving of oneself'. Gilbert Ryle[4] famously distinguished between 'knowing that' and 'knowing how' – the knowledge of the kinds of factual or theoretical propositions one might find in books, on the one hand, and 'practical capability' – having the expertise to accomplish sometimes very demanding things (for example, advance projects, tackle problems, help people feel less insecure, etc.) in real-world contexts on the other. Both are manifested and needed here. Expertise, in this broader sense, is thus very closely related to those accounts of professionalism that focus on an indicative list of admirable dispositions or 'virtues', saying, for example, that a nurse who exercises professionalism will embody qualities such as theoretical understanding, practical competence and thoroughness, compassion, honesty, courage, fairness, integrity (or similar virtues). Lists like this, often accompanied by reference to general principles, and sometimes also by more focused and specific lists of 'dos and don'ts' or 'shoulds and musts', also crop up in codes of ethics that are often treated as a defining feature of a professional group.

Professionalism in this sense – of embodied admirable qualities – thus holds together the person of the professional, their expertise and their ethics. But these things are not just accidentally parcelled up together; rather, they are closely interconnected. Up until now, we have tended to talk about 'technical standards' and 'ethical standards' as if these necessarily picked out different things. The former might be thought to refer to the correct application of specialist knowledge and the latter to the correct comportment of professionals in social space – what we called relational expertise at the end of chapter 3 – and the ways in which they navigate the practice dilemmas they face. However, in the case of Helen, it is evident that these things will for the most part be practised together and that there are many matters which seem to sit between, or cut across, the two. (Furthermore – as we will argue next – there are fundamental conceptual connections between these two dimensions.) There are some concerns that Helen deals with that have a large and inherently technical aspect – such as the dosage and administration of drugs – but any judgements that Helen makes about these things always take place in social and ethical space, and in negotiation with others (including family members) and involve the weighing up of other people's (professional and lay) opinions, values and preferences and not just 'scientific' factors. In addition, many of the judgements Helen has to make – such as when to go round to the family home – are not 'technical' in this narrow scientific sense, but are experience-based practical judgements about both the clinical and socio-emotional salience of what is being said to her. These are judgements that draw upon her as a person and on her 'humanity', not just her knowledge in an impersonal sense.

Expertise and ethics are connected at a fundamental level; *to have expertise* – at least in this arena of health and social care but arguably in general – *is to have additional (i.e. non-universal) personal resources to do some good.* By definition, valuable 'know-how' is knowing how to do something well. If the 'something' is at all worthwhile, and not wholly private and/or pointless (like being able to wiggle one's ears), then an intrinsic part of doing something well involves having regard both for the potentially good ends that are at stake and the ethical balancing acts that are involved in pursuing and attaining those goods. The kind of expertise that is sought after and socially recognized in professionals such as Helen certainly falls into this category.

Pulling things together: professionalism as expertise-based social authority

The idea of professionalism as expertise-based social authority joins these two dimensions together. The ideal type suggested is one in which a professional group has specialized know-how and a significant degree of resulting and licensed social influence in specific domains such that they can exercise that know-how, including the relevant ethical dispositions, to promote the good ends towards which the expertise is directed. These two dimensions reflect the crux of the 'trait theories' and lists of traits discussed in chapter 2 – including both the ones that stress the qualities of professional practitioners and those that stress the social recognition of and properties of professions. These two dimensions have also sometimes been linked by the relationship between two senses of 'authority' – i.e. someone is 'an authority' when they have expertise that is worth acting upon; and someone is 'in authority' when they are in a position, and have recognized social 'powers', to make things happen in certain spheres.[5] Helen and her colleagues fulfil both these linked conditions and this combination is what is embedded in the idea of professionalism that we are elaborating upon here.

In order for professionalism to be possible and to be practised on this account, a lot of conditions have to be met. These conditions include suitable social, political and institutional arrangements and suitable personal and interpersonal dispositions and relationships. Aspirations towards professionalism can 'fail' because occupational groups and individuals are denied the autonomy and scope for licensed social influence that is required; or they can fail because individual practitioners fall short, in general or on specific occasions, in relation to the expertise and broader admirable qualities that are deemed necessary to serve the ends of the profession. These are different kinds of judgements – the first refers to the 'social possibility' of someone exercising professionalism; the second refers to whether an individual (or team, unit, etc.) fails or succeeds in realizing this possibility. Of course, these sets of conditions are being discussed in relation to an ideal type, but in reality the conditions will typically fall far short of ideal. In practice, we should think of these judgements as a matter of degree but also have in mind that there may be a minimum threshold of both licensed social influence and relevant capabilities and dispositions below which we might say it does not really make sense to talk about professionalism in the sense we are outlining here.

How does this account relate to the grounds for scepticism reviewed in chapter 3? We would suggest that the two pictures – the sceptical picture sketched in the previous chapter and the ideal type outlined above are broadly compatible with one another. Some of the scepticism relates to whether professionalism is 'socially possible' in certain climates and cases. This seems to be a very important question to which the answer is often far from clear. We told the story of Helen's service in a way that assumes it is possible, but it is easy to imagine real-world pressures or reforms of her service conditions which would make one doubt this assumption. Some of the scepticism relates to whether the kind of personal devotion or commitment (and allied ethical conscientiousness) is available in contemporary conditions – whether professionalism is 'personally possible'. Again, this seems to be an important point and one that, in our brief portrait, Helen worries about for herself. Finally, some of the scepticism relates to *critiques* of professionalism – reflected, for example, in the argument that professionalism can be responsible for bad as well as good. As indicated at the start of this chapter (using the analogy of friendship), we would suggest that these two things – the good and the bad – can coexist and that it is a mistake to uncritically celebrate professionalism or any other value or set of social practices.

To some, it may seem contradictory to say that we should recognize professionalism as an important good and at the same time acknowledge the strength of the critiques that have been made of professionalism – that it might, for example, be exclusionary, reinforce unnecessary hierarchies and, in some cases, be associated with a foolish or vain preoccupation with social status. But we would argue that it is not a contradiction at all. The easiest way to imagine this, we suggest, is to differentiate between evaluating things in 'ideal' and 'non-ideal' circumstances. In an ideal world, for example, there might be no need for 'judges' or 'ombudsmen'. People would not harm one another or would resolve their disputes or repair their relationships through mutually respectful dialogue. Similarly, in an ideal world everyone's expertise could be brought to bear, and balanced, appropriately and effectively in decision-making and in collective processes of social coordination. All socially 'authoritative' roles and institutions may be viewed by some people not only as less desirable and less sensitive than an ideal alternative, but also as having significant side effects that need to be critiqued. On the other hand, in the non-ideal circumstances that make up the 'real world', many of these same people might accept that these roles and institutions have a valuable place. Specifically, as indicated above, if all social organization in a domain where context-sensitive expertise is relevant was dominated by market or bureaucratic pressures in ways that were unresponsive to expertise, the same people might arguably see a vital role for forms of professionalism.

What professionalism demands

The line we want to pursue here (and which we will follow for the remainder of the book) is: first, that there remains something important and desirable about the abstract conception of professionalism we have just outlined; second, that something approximating this conception is also still a practical possibility, at least in some cases and circumstances, but that it is difficult to realize both socially and personally; and third, that enactment of professionalism is, therefore, a demanding social and personal exercise. In particular, we want to stress that what makes it demanding does not relate just to the level of technical difficulty or abstract specialization, but it involves individual and collective agents working (and sometimes struggling) to deliver on the necessary conditions and activities, and doing so in ways that depend upon practical, political and ethical judgements and emotional and human resources (in other words, what we have crudely labelled as 'relational expertise' as well as technical expertise). We will say a little bit more about each of these things in this concluding section and this will also enable us to say something about the relationship between the two senses of 'ideal' with which we began – the abstract model or ideal type of professionalism that we have summarized and the personal ideals (values, virtues and visions) of practitioners.

The quest for professionalism has to be seen as an inherently political as well as an ethical one. It necessarily involves struggles over how society is organized (because other modes of social coordination are very strong); and it involves professionals being ready to see their work in the context of broader debates about social and civic purposes. It is worth noting that this expansive conception of professionalism is either disguised by, or is different from, some of the ways in which professionalism is more routinely talked about.

Some of the dominant discourses around professionalism in, for example, educational and other policy contexts, stress narrow and neutral-sounding ideas. This is (perhaps best) seen in the language of 'skills' or 'competences'. Such very general constructions of the knowledge base of practitioners not only fudge and 'flatten out' the great variation in the kinds of knowledge and purposes manifested in complex occupations, but they cover up the inherently ethical and political nature of professional roles. Even when values are acknowledged, and something like 'admirable dispositions' are directly or indirectly referred to, this is often done in a similarly neutral manner, using the language of 'attitudes' – a language which foregrounds individuals' psychology as manifest in overt behaviours, rather than in questions about character and social purpose.[6] This kind of neutral language lends itself to, and reinforces, both the 'what works' emphasis of the evidence-based movement and the 'tick-box' forms of accountability and performance management that prevail in organizational models of professionalism.

In reality, we would suggest, these technicist and managerial emphases should themselves be seen as value-systems or ideologies; but they are ones that reduce and 'tame' the potential of professionalism in the richer sense we want to defend. Professionalism in the sense we have outlined involves being routinely reflexive and self-critical, and this includes being ready to challenge managerial and organizational norms; it also involves being ready to play an active role in redefining these norms and being prepared to work both inside and outside employing organizations to help shape the broader social landscape. This is not to suggest that professionals should always see themselves in combative or antagonistic relationships with their employing institutions or engaged in overt politics or activism – only that these possibilities need to be embraced within a full conception of professionalism. This should be clear if we think about the professionals who make up the paediatric oncology outreach service that we have used as our example in this chapter. It may be that these practitioners (or practitioners in similar services) are happy with the way in which the NHS and other agencies support and organize their work, and feel that there is sufficient recognition given to their own and their clients' contributions in co-designing and delivering these services. In such cases, there would be a rough correspondence between managerial (and other institutional) arrangements and professional perspectives – with the former harnessing the latter effectively. But if this were not the case, then we would think it legitimate, and perhaps even a professional duty, for the practitioners concerned to lobby for better services for the people who they judge are being poorly served. Similarly, these practitioners may need to be ready to argue for a redrawing or realignment of professional or institutional boundaries as part of that process. This might well put such practitioners in an uncomfortable position with their employers or colleagues and involve them in making difficult strategic and tactical choices about how most effectively to intervene (there are costs and benefits to both more combative and more conciliatory modes of influence). But all we are arguing here is that such tricky ethical and political dilemmas should properly be seen as falling within rather than outside the remit of professional ethics.

We obviously do not want to suggest that there is only one proper set of ideals or mode of being for a would-be professional – that, for example, he or she should be committed to a particular ideological stance. There must be scope for different kinds of political and practical emphases. However, we are saying that professionalism in the ideal-type sense is necessarily connected to practitioner ideals of some sort. This is because, to repeat, the notion of licensed expertise that underpins professionalism contains within it an orientation towards social purposes and a responsibility for making difficult discriminations about what is for the best in general or in response to specific practice dilemmas. The virtues of a professional are, thus, necessarily broad-ranging. There is an extremely important place for what might be thought of as undramatic workaday virtues – turning up on time and consistently applying one's skills. In addition, in many cases, even routine work in health and social care involves more than just following a script; it requires balancing different, and sometimes competing, values and interests, and calls, for example, on the classical virtues of practical wisdom, temperance, justice and courage. Professionalism cannot be practised simply by applying value-free, technically defined, authoritatively prescribed competences – because such things, in so far as they make sense and are possible at all, will simply not do the job. Sometimes the kinds of judgement called for exceed the 'routine' complex balancing acts required in immediate day-to-day practice, involving questions about society and politics more broadly. Such judgements might relate to the role of one's professional organization, and/or the broader contribution made by, and constraints placed upon, one's professional group, and/or social and political debates about purposes, priorities, systems and cultures that affect one's ability to make a contribution or, more generally, pose a threat to the goods and services one has expertise about. This broader social orientation calls for civic virtues as well as practice virtues – the readiness and capability to be a good citizen at least locally, and sometimes more widely. All of this follows from the insight that professionalism is a mode of social coordination. In short, one of the tasks of professionals is to help deliver and defend certain models of social organization and decision-making over others.

The need for a measure of ideological literacy and civic virtue is just one illustration of how the intellectual qualities needed for professionalism stretch beyond the capabilities associated with specific technical, professional or academic disciplines. Health and social care practitioners often need the literacy to find out about, understand or apply relevant 'evidence' claims. But, if they are to do this skilfully and in a way that is responsive to the multiple contingencies and controversies embedded in practice, they also need to be able to question the bases of the knowledge claims and to have the broader critical capacity to assess the relevance of these knowledge claims in the context of other considerations, including those of value and purpose. Ideally, this critical capacity will be fuelled both by intellectual curiosity and openness to competing theories, including both rival scientific theories and other kinds of relevant theoretical perspectives, for example from the social sciences and humanities. Those who possess this broad range of intellectual capability – and we readily admit that this is rather an exacting and idealized characterization – are likely to combine both confidence and humility in the way they approach their work. They will be relatively confident in those areas where they draw on substantial expertise and experience, whilst at the same time recognizing not only the limits of their expertise but the ever-present possibility that they are missing an important part of the picture. Of course, it should not be forgotten that some of the expertise central to doing a good job is scientific or technical and is itself constantly evolving – and so even keeping up with this dimension of knowledge is potentially demanding work. For example, Helen and colleagues need to be ready to learn about new treatment modalities or information technology developments, such as long-distance clinical monitoring or virtual meetings. Nonetheless, if practitioners only engage with such developments as passive 'knowledge consumers' and not as critical learners, with at least one eye on protecting the experiences of the families they care for, the benefits to them, their clients and to the quality of service provision will be much smaller.

What this discussion of civic and intellectual virtues shows is that, in talking about the qualities needed for professionalism, we are necessarily talking about people's motivations and dispositions, and this includes talking about their emotional lives. Furthermore, as is evident from the example of Helen discussed above, working in health and social care often has a direct emotional component; that is, it is not just work that is 'accompanied by' emotions but is often work that involves focusing on or more or less deliberately working with and through emotions. There are various literatures that have addressed this area and these show the inherent complexities of emotional issues and the costs and benefits of addressing them. For example, there is classic work in nursing on the way in which practitioners of care systems can defend themselves from destabilizing emotional threats which risk not only cutting them off from patients who are in need of more substantial forms of communication and contact, but also from ways of properly addressing their own anxieties.[7] There is extensive and parallel discussion about the benefits and risks of the 'emotional neutrality' in the hidden curriculum of medical education and of the difficulty of combining the scientific and professional detachment needed for sound technical judgement with the sensitivity and personal openness that is needed for effective empathy and compassion.[8] There is also widely cited literature on 'emotional labour' (most commonly related to the nursing role but now applied much more extensively), which seeks to acknowledge and positively articulate the work practitioners like Helen do to contain, support and 'manage' their own and their clients' feelings.[9] Helen's work, for example, is a good illustration of the unavoidable challenge of managing social distance. On the one hand, the work involves profoundly closing down the distance between 'professional' and 'client' to allow for a proper meeting of the people involved. But, for very good reasons, this cannot justify calling for a simple and ever-increasing dissolution of distance. Professionals have not only to protect themselves emotionally, but they have also to be ready, when necessary, to play the part of trustworthy guide or authority figure, and they have forms of accountability that extend wider than the immediate patient or family with whom they are dealing.

Although the degree and kind of emotion work clearly varies across roles, settings and different cases, practitioners often have to combine a degree of attentiveness and responsiveness to their own and other people's feelings (for example, to the anger, resentment, resignation, despair, grief, etc. of the people they are dealing with) with the practical robustness and resilience to provide ongoing advice, support and access to service resources, even when these may be unwelcome or may seem in some respects 'besides the point'. This combination of sensitivity and practical support clearly has the potential to be extremely stressful and to exert a substantial emotional burden on practitioners themselves. Good services will recognize this fact and will provide mechanisms of professional support that help relieve the burden, in part through enabling individuals to develop insight into the causes and manifestations of the stress they experience. Nonetheless, as with intellectual resources, the emotional resources needed to exercise professionalism are potentially extremely demanding.

Conclusion

Given the broad picture we have sketched here, the nature of professionalism as both a social and individual accomplishment becomes clearer. Professionalism at an individual level does not become possible unless and until professional roles are socially supported. This means that social influence and coordination based upon professional expertise have not only to be 'allowed' in climates where market or bureaucratic power may be considerable, but also to be institutionally organized and underpinned. This makes professionalism at an individual level a possibility. However, this is only a starting point for individual practitioners. Although practitioners can and ought to be able to derive moral and intellectual support from the professional groups and teams they belong to, they also need to be able to summon up the personal resources to exercise professionalism 'on their own'. As we have outlined in this chapter, this is often no easy task and requires intellectual, ethical, civic and emotional capacities and know-how. No doubt this is as it should be. We can hardly license individuals to exercise expertise-based social influence without placing high expectations on them. Both social and personal resources are central to professionalism. This is why – as illustrated in chapter 2 – some accounts of professional 'traits' emphasize social and institutional conditions (for example, knowledge base, professional organization, threshold of collective autonomy) and some emphasize the desirable qualities of practitioners (for example, integrity, service or altruistic stance, threshold of individual autonomy). This is also why a claim to professionalism might be seen as a claim to be 'special' in two different ways – as occupying a socially recognized position of influence and as embodying the qualities needed to fulfil the demands of such a position. Professionalism, we might say in summary, depends upon a combination of personal qualities and achievements and specific forms of social organization – it is the accomplished exercise of expertise-based social authority.

Of course, this chapter has been about an ideal type and some associated ideals. In practice, necessarily imperfect social conditions and normal human frailty mean that individuals and groups will sometimes fall short of these ideals. Furthermore, there will be interactions between these two things. Where social and institutional conditions fall short, it becomes less reasonable to ask so much from individuals. Where individuals do accomplish high levels of professionalism in adverse circumstances, this is likely to be at very high cost to themselves. And where individuals positively fall short of decent levels of working and caring, this may partly be because they have been 'let down' by the systems they work in. Ultimately, however, and of course, individuals cannot be exempted from a measure of responsibility for the things they do. In the remaining chapters, we will focus on the challenges of enacting professionalism both individually and socially. We will focus on what might broadly be characterized as the ethical challenges, but, as we have tried to show, these cannot be neatly separated from intellectual, civic and emotional challenges.

CHAPTER FIVE

Integrity at Work

Professionalism, for individual practitioners, involves finding a way to navigate through turbulent waters and to negotiate cross-currents. It is impossible to be a good professional without being able to live with, and somehow handle, difficult judgements including dilemmas. The notion of 'dilemmas' might, for some, conjure up unusual and dramatic situations in which individuals wrestle with themselves and others emotionally and intellectually. These situations are certainly a part of professional life but, in this chapter, we use the idea of dilemmas in a more wide-ranging way to encompass not just 'turbulent waters' but also many kinds of 'cross-currents' – all those situations in which professionals are, for good reasons, pushed or pulled in different directions. These latter may not always be particularly dramatic, indeed may not even be consciously brought to mind or deliberated about. But they still involve practitioners in finding a path where more than one seems desirable. If practitioners are to conscientiously find the right path, they will need to draw upon the intellectual and ethical virtues discussed in the previous chapter. A professional code of ethics may act as a broad guide here but will be insufficient for coping with day-to-day detail and variations. In addition, practitioners must be ready to continuously develop, apply and test their own ethical compass against their professional experience. In short, they must be ready to practise integrity in their work.

The possibility of tensions between different kinds of concerns and values, as we have indicated in various places in previous chapters, is inherent in professionalism. Dilemmas are not merely added complications that professionals may encounter – although they may be these too – but they are built into professional roles. We have seen this, for example, in relation to the two facets of 'new professionalism' that urge health and social care professionals to work in partnership with clients and, at the same time, specify care standards. Can professionals both be responsive to service users' preferences and provide the care that is deemed good (according to standardized norms), and what should they do if and when these conflict? But even without focusing on models of new professionalism, it is possible to see analogous, and fundamental, tensions in the very idea of professional roles. In very general and simplified terms, we can see this as the broad tension between constructions of professionals as, on the one hand, 'powerful experts' and, on the other, as 'supporters or carers'. This tension can take many different forms and can be presented in multiple ways, seen from different perspectives and with different emphases. In some respects, it echoes the distinction between critical and idealistic readings of professionalism. As we have noted (in chapter 2), some sociological readings of professionalism see these different emphases as 'joined together' in ideologies of professionalization. Professionalization projects are, at one and the same time, oriented towards social status and influence and towards service and the promotion of good – it is not a case of 'either/or' but of 'both/and'. Health and social care professionals are meant, at least to some extent, to be both 'social legislators' and 'social servants' – their role should enable them to help shape social organization within specific domains and require them to be responsive to the needs, and attuned to the good, of those for whom they aspire to work. The position of service users or clients is also complex and unstable. Although recent changes in social and policy climates tend to be summarized as a shift of service users from passive to active, the reality is more complicated. As Clarke and Newman put it:

> It is the new 'common sense' that public service users have shifted from the deferential to the assertive; from the ignorant to the knowledgeable; from the passive to the active voice – in short, from citizens to consumers. But such shifts are profoundly uneven . . . They may be distributed between different sorts of people; but people are themselves neither stable nor unitary in their encounters with services. The same person may combine being a knowledgeable expert of their own condition; a rights bearing and assertive citizen; an anxious dependent and a seeker after professional help and advice across a series of encounters with the health service.[1]

Whilst starting this chapter by acknowledging this very general underlying tension between the 'assertive' and the 'responsive' elements of professionalism, we definitely do not want to give the impression that value judgements in professionalism can be reduced to this one giant dilemma or balancing act. The real situation is hugely complicated and requires the elucidation of many different sorts of dilemmas and tensions, and an understanding of how they intersect with one another in ever varying mixtures across different contexts and cases. Even a superficial awareness of the famous four principles of ethics[2] – non-maleficence, beneficence, respect for autonomy and justice – can be used to start to fill out some of this complexity. Practitioners, if they wish to be able to offer an ethical defence for what they do, need, at the very least, to have some recognition that their expert 'interference' in a situation can do harm as well as good, and some account of how and why they think the latter might 'offset' the former. Similarly, they will need an awareness that respecting the autonomy of individuals, by trying to respond to their wishes and preferences, is not only potentially in conflict with beneficence to that individual, but may also exact some 'cost' on wider groups or populations – and thus may be in tension with other important concerns such as social justice or population-level effectiveness. The more we focus in on the different value conflicts that can arise, and the more we look at specific cases, the more complicated things become.

In the remainder of this chapter, we will make use of a few examples to illustrate some of the dilemmas that health and social care professionals face. We will make no attempt to capture the full range of these dilemmas – this would be an enormous task and is not part of our purpose here – but rather we will use these examples to consider the challenges of professional judgement and the implications these present for successfully occupying a professional role. Some of the issues that arise will be more related to the question of designing and supporting professional roles than to the business of occupying them, and we will follow these up more fully in the next chapter. We hope the chapter will help illuminate some of the characteristic balancing acts that arise across professional roles in health and social care. In particular, we have in mind – as well as the broad background balance between the 'assertive' and 'responsive' dimensions of professionalism introduced above – balances between serving individual and collective goods, and between the agency of individual practitioners and the collective agency of the services they work within. We will conclude the chapter by reflecting on one of the core challenges of enacting professionalism: exercising a degree of social power with integrity.

An example

Saira is a health visitor.[3] She has called in to see Telesia and her new baby boy, Luca. Saira knows that Telesia struggled, and failed, to give up smoking completely during her pregnancy and is concerned that she may revert to heavy smoking now that Luca has been born. She arrives with this thought in mind and the intention of reinforcing the message about the advantages of giving up and the offer of smoking cessation support. However, on arrival she finds that Telesia is rather overwhelmed by her immediate life circumstances – she is facing accommodation problems, is generally struggling to make ends meet and is very short of sleep. Saira does some routine checks on Luca, tries to offer advice, contacts, suggestions and reassurance on some of Telesia's problems but decides not to broach the smoking-related advice. On the way to her next visit, Saira still feels that she did the right thing; but she is not completely sure – perhaps, she wonders, she is too quick to 'go with the flow' and might have done much more good for Telesia and Luca by not changing course.

This is an example of a fairly routine and 'non-dramatic' professional judgement. Saira does not experience her judgement as involving a significant dilemma but, as we have summarized it here, she does have some sense of tension between two courses of action – the one she had originally envisaged and the one she actually took – and is left with a 'question mark' about whether she did the right thing. It is worth highlighting this element of uncertainty and the accompanying cognitive and emotional load generated even in such a routine and unproblematic case because this reminds us that – when considered cumulatively and given the much more substantial dilemmas that sometimes arise – there is a potentially high burden attached to professional judgement.

The ethical tensions in the work of health visitors, including examples of this kind, are illustrated and analysed in more depth by Julie Greenway and colleagues.[4] Their account is very helpful and we will draw upon it as we bring some more elements and dimensions of this example into view. Greenway et al. show (through the analysis of qualitative interviews) that health visitors find themselves in this kind of situation comparatively frequently. On another occasion, it may be a discussion about breastfeeding, or some other professional concern, that is (at least temporarily) set aside. In many instances, a conversation based upon some professional agenda (such as in the smoking case) is started but it just does not get very far because the client quickly blocks it or makes it clear that they really do not wish to engage with it. Whether or not the conversation is dropped in anticipation or whilst in progress, there are a variety of ways in which the potential tension might be described – and the best account will probably involve a combination of these descriptions and will vary from case to case. First, it could be seen as a tension between different professional constructions of the client's needs and priorities – the professional could simply judge that x is, at least for now, less important than y. Second, it could be seen as a tension between what the professional judges to be important and what the client judges to be important – and thus an example of the tension between beneficence and respect for autonomy. Third, it could be seen as a tension between what is desirable and what is realistic – that is, that it would in one sense be right to promote smoking cessation but it is very unlikely to work and so, for that reason, it is not a sensible thing to pursue and might, in reality, cause only unproductive upset.

Greenway et al.'s account also adds in other layers of readings which merit consideration. For example, health visitors point to the central importance of 'relationship building' and trust in their work with clients and, therefore, to the importance – whether for intrinsic or instrumental reasons – of privileging the more open-ended long-term relationship over some short-term professionally prescribed and focused intervention. This is a recognizable concern in our everyday life and the ways in which anyone interacts with their friends and colleagues. We value other people and the relationships that we have with them and sometimes suspend our prior agendas because these seem to intrude into, or risk undermining, the relationship. Although the practice may look much the same, there is clearly a difference in principle between sustaining relationships for intrinsic reasons and sustaining them for instrumental reasons. Greenway et al.'s data show elements of both. Health visitors are there to do a job (to protect and promote families' health and well-being) and so there is absolutely nothing inherently wrong with them acting in part for instrumental reasons – the trust they foster enables them to do their job in the longer term. However, there is also an element of them doing their job *through* the very act of building relationships and trust – these things can be seen as valuable ends in themselves, providing part of the climate that enables clients to feel supported and able to manage.

Greenway et al.'s analysis also illuminates other factors relating to the broader context of health-visiting work that need to be taken into account. In particular, they highlight two overlapping considerations. First, health visitors are expected to make a contribution to population health and to deliver on wider service targets relating to public health, and this can lead to tensions between population goals and the needs and concerns of individual clients. Second, these kinds of public health targets are just one example of a wider set of organizational drivers that shape the expectations we have of health visitors. Health visitors cannot simply determine their own role and tasks for themselves. As well as reflecting substantive tensions, such as the one between population level and individual level well-being, these organizational drivers can create tensions between institutional or managerial demands and health visitors' own sense of purpose and priorities. We will further explore the importance of these two considerations in the two subsequent sections of this chapter.

Thus even this relatively mundane and non-controversial example illustrates the pervasiveness of value judgements facing all health and social care professionals. Some of the tensions involved may be seen as pragmatic rather than ethical ones (for example, we might think that Saira is wholly right to pursue the smoking cessation advice, even if it is unwelcome, but tactically wise to pick her time); but even many of these can be reframed as dilemmas of professional ethics. As well as 'trademark' ethical issues such as the tensions between autonomy and beneficence or justice there are: (1) broader questions about professional ideals and purposes, for example: What is the crux of what I am trying to do? How far should I be population-focused or client-focused in my practice? What aspects of health and well-being should I be focusing on and when am I straying beyond either professional or personal boundaries? And (2) specific issues about professional comportment, for example – how far and where is it legitimate for me to remain quiet about, or even disguise, some of my own or my organization's professional agendas? How far do I owe openness, and an element of authenticity, to my clients or are these sometimes unaffordable luxuries?

There are strong parallels between the situation that Saira finds herself in and that of other health and social care professionals, although there are, of course, also areas of potential difference which we will come back to later. All health and social care professionals have to find ways of steering through a landscape of value tensions and cross-currents – both routinely and sometimes in heightened ways – concerning purposes, priorities, principles and pragmatism. Similarly, they will, more or less frequently – partly depending on their character – find themselves reflecting on, and worrying about, their personal and professional integrity, whether and when they are doing the right thing. As a practitioner, it is often difficult to feel wholly comfortable about one's decisions and practices because one is inevitably balancing multiple, and sometimes conflicting, considerations – and often having to do so 'on the spot' by relying on one's accumulated experience and insight – a process that is very likely to generate a sense that one is failing in some respect or other.

In this situation, concerns about one's integrity are very rarely going to be met by the judgement that every possible 'good end' has been served and every possible 'bad end' has been avoided. Rather, the highest aspiration can only be to manage the various ethical and practical tensions to the best of one's ability on the basis of one's conscientious ethical judgement. Integrity in this sense involves striving towards a coherent ethical vision and practice, but it also includes being ready to live with some elements of incoherence and untidiness. In the next two sections of this chapter, we explore some of the challenges to integrity further by returning to two of the broad themes identified in Greenway et al.'s analysis which also have relevance to many other professional roles.

Collective good or individual good?

The tensions built into health-visiting roles between public-health-facing and client-facing emphases also apply to other roles. It is most conspicuous in primary healthcare and community roles but, from time to time, it has clear relevance to all roles (because, for example, any professional may have to deal with clients who, in one way or another, constitute a potential risk to the well-being of others). These tensions also have widespread relevance because of the many ways that changing policy contexts can change the relationships that practitioners have with service users. For example, when something comes to be labelled as a public health priority – such as alcohol use, teenage pregnancy, communicable diseases – it often becomes a focus of new funding and practice initiatives (and sometimes targets) which, in turn, can shape all manner of established and new roles. One illustration of this is the way in which the UK National Teenage Pregnancy Strategy created new tensions for an established and new workforce, including social and youth workers, who were encouraged to combine biomedically and politically inspired concerns about the reduction of teenage pregnancy rates at a population level with an orientation towards the non-judgemental acceptance of, and support for, individual teenage mothers.[5] Once again, this example shows how the conflicts in this kind of situation are often twofold. It is not just that practitioners may be pushed or pulled in different directions by different emphases, but also that they may feel a dissonance between their own conceptions of 'what matters' and the 'official' conceptions that are shaping their role descriptions.

Public health is, of course, only one way of conceiving of 'collective goods' – that which is good for groups, communities or populations. There are very many potential tensions for professionals who need to face 'both ways', towards the individual in front of them and towards the good of society; and there are a range of different dimensions and interpretations of both of these things. It may be worth emphasizing again that these kinds of tension are built into professional roles. On the one hand, professionals exist to serve some good (and goods cannot be wholly reduced to individuals) and, at the very least, they have obligations to monitor and limit the harmful social side effects of their work. On the other hand, professionals typically have a specific set of clients or service users with whom they have significant relationships and to whom they have special obligations. (Although, of course, the centre of gravity of different professional roles will vary, with some relatively more client-focused and some relatively more population-focused.)

Sarah Banks's overview of ethics in social work, for example, shows how this tension is never far from the surface in the professional lives of social workers and also provides a helpful account of the complexities lying behind a simple-sounding idea like 'collective good' and how substantial and knotty the associated dilemmas can be.[6] Banks's fourfold taxonomy of ethical concerns in social work includes two sets of concerns that we have already touched upon and that often centre on the professional–client dyad. These relate to the tensions between autonomy and beneficence and worries about ethically appropriate relationships and boundaries. Her taxonomy also includes two sets of concerns that intrinsically relate to our current theme – the social ends of social work – which she labels as issues related to 'public welfare' and issues related to 'equality, difference and structural oppression'.

It is also worth briefly summarizing the two examples she offers to illustrate these concerns. In relation to the first, she uses a case in which social workers are asked to work with the police to help them catch a sexually exploitative middle-aged man who is in a relationship with, and appears to be preying upon, one of their clients (a twelve-year-old girl in a residential care home). They have willingly placed restrictions on the movement of the girl; but should they cooperate in a plan which involves the girl being allowed to make meeting arrangements with the man in order for the police to catch him? In relation to the second, she uses the example of a drop-in centre in rural Wales that has been working hard to ensure it is accessible to, and used by, the local young men of Bangladeshi and Muslim heritage. This policy is successful until families become aware of the sexual health provision and advice aspects of the centre and a community meeting held at the local Mosque determines that these young men should not be allowed to use the drop-in centre unless and until this aspect of its work is dropped. Banks presents this as a long-standing and deep-seated conflict: the providers are committed to social inclusion in their work (as well as to meeting the individual entitlements of young people), but also see inclusion as involving sensitivity towards and respect for the different values of user groups.

These are good examples of the less routine and more 'dramatic' kinds of dilemmas that face health and social care professionals. They each open up a range of complications and help to illustrate the intractability of some dilemmas. Unlike the example concerning Saira – which just involved a small perturbation in the rhythm of her work and thoughts – these are cases where uncertainties about 'doing the right thing' are not only likely to be much greater but are likely to generate interpersonal and social conflict both between different social workers (with different value commitments) and between social workers and others. These kinds of dilemmas are not just intellectual puzzles, but they carry a powerful emotional charge and may generate anger, frustration, resentment, disillusionment and so on. Managing them – especially in an

environment where one's workload is intensifying, as discussed in the previous chapter – is hugely demanding. Having
acknowledged this, however, it is also important to recognize
what we have called elsewhere 'routine moral stress';[7] that is,
the more 'low-level' and pervasive tensions between different potential purposes and priorities which are a continuous
feature of professional work. These low-level tensions are, in
many ways, of equal importance to understanding the challenges of professionalism. Their importance arises from
their relative invisibility. Dramatic cases have the 'advantage'
of bringing value disputes to the surface. By contrast, practitioners like Saira are constantly adopting positions about
'low-level' issues, thereby helping to determine or reinforce
the ethical orientation of their profession without, sometimes,
even noticing that this is what is going on.

Banks's use of the label 'equality, difference and structural
oppression' as part of her typology (designed to reflect the
concerns of social workers themselves) is worth noting. Social
work is oriented towards social, as well as personal, ends and
necessitates an orientation and sensitivity towards cultural
and political issues – for example, working in conjunction
with people in social movements or activist groups. For that
reason, social workers will often be particularly attuned to
critical agendas and may have an active interest in debates
about different conceptions of social justice, identity politics
and so on.[8] This typology and Banks's examples thereby also
illustrate the potential for professionals in different areas to
learn from one another. The complexities of conceptualizing
equality and of respecting difference, and the ways in which
individuals and groups can find themselves excluded, dis-
advantaged and damaged by institutions and broader social
structures (independently of the intentions of individuals),
are important factors in all sectors and roles but are not always
clearly signalled or articulated.

The language of 'ethics' used within mainstream healthcare professions tends to omit or 'smooth over' these more

critical or politicized readings (although their relevance and huge importance is recognized and treated within the sociology of healthcare literature). One area where identity politics and the importance of 'voice' have, however, become influential in mainstream healthcare policy concerns the recognition of patients and families as key stakeholders and agents in the healthcare system. There is now a near-universal expectation that 'patient voice' should somehow play a part in key decisions about planning or evaluating healthcare services and research. This encompasses not only the inclusion of patient representatives or lay expertise in professional decision-making fora, but also increasingly an important place at the policy table for autonomously organized patient groups.[9]

Control and autonomy in professional roles

Without rehearsing any of the other countless examples that could be cited to illustrate professional dilemmas, the challenges of professional judgement are already evident. However, as indicated in the account above, there is another crucial dimension of maintaining integrity in professional work. How far are the judgements that are exercised actually the judgements of individual practitioners (acting separately or cooperatively) and how far are they determined by policies, organizations and managers and, to some extent or other, imposed upon practitioners? How can a practitioner reconcile what they personally judge to be the right thing to do with what they are 'told' is the right thing to do?

In a climate of 'organizational professionalism', this is a question of fundamental importance. The health visitors that Greenway et al. studied were concerned that the targets they were given not only made them liable to be less responsive (and of less value) to their clients but, by their nature – through the way the targets partly defined and performance-managed their roles – undermined their own professional judgement and capacity for professionalism.

There are at least three ways in which this practical and ethical tension – between organizational and personal values – can be analysed. One possibility is to say that if an occupational role is substantially 'managed', and subject to more or less forceful controls, then it fails to qualify as, or ceases to be, a professional role at all – that professionalism depends upon substantial levels of practitioner autonomy. On this interpretation, the challenge for practitioners aspiring to professionalism – as well as to do their jobs to the best of their abilities – is to struggle against the conditions of their work and to seek to lessen the degree of prescriptive organizational control over their day-to-day judgements. In other words, it is to pursue 'professionalization projects' in their work. Another possibility is for practitioners to seek to 'work around', resist or subvert official organizational expectations – to attempt to preserve a large area of autonomy and discretion whilst paying 'lip-service' to organizational targets and ticking the necessary bureaucratic boxes. This is not an easy position. It will sometimes be impossible to conform to both one's sense of vocation and one's institutional responsibilities, and it not only introduces dissonance into the role but also involves, to some extent, doing one's job twice, or with 'two heads'. A third possibility is to accept that all professional roles will involve a balance between organizational control and practitioner autonomy and to see an awareness of this fact, and the skill of managing it, as part of professionalism properly understood. Some combination of these ways of understanding and approaching this tension probably makes sense.

The challenge of having to manage the hybrid identity of being both an organizational agent and at the same time an individually accountable worker – indeed, of having to sometimes wear multiple 'hats' – is common to all professional roles. Once again it is, for example, well recognized and articulated in the field of social work where an international statement on ethical principles begins by underlining the nature of the dilemmatic terrain on which social workers operate, in particular:

- the fact that the loyalty of social workers is often in the middle of conflicting interests;
- the fact that social workers operate both as helpers and controllers;
- the conflicts between the duty of social workers to protect the interest of people with whom they work and societal demands for efficiency and utility;
- the fact that resources in society are limited.[10]

Enacting professionalism on this sort of terrain involves finding the right balance between 'being controlled' and 'being autonomous'. This in turn depends, of course, on the case in hand and also upon empirical questions (what exactly are the kinds of organizational control in place?) and interpretive or ideological questions (what kinds of, and how much, professional autonomy do we deem necessary for something to be a professional role?). But two things are clear: first, the health and social care professions, including that most traditional and powerful profession of medicine, have been subject to increasing degrees of organizational control in recent decades; second, however much these kinds of controls are reined back or moderated in the future, there will always be some element of organizational control in place. It is the nature of professional work that it is governed, coordinated and harnessed by social institutions. A completely free-floating and 'wholly self-directed' professional – even if this possibility made sense – would not be a professional at all. Part of the challenge of steering a course through professional work is combining and striking a balance between one's own interpretations of one's purposes and priorities and the official interpretations that govern or manage one's work – in short, between vocational and institutional identities. Leaning too much towards the former can risk making oneself an unreliable, professionally unaccountable and potentially self-indulgent practitioner.

Leaning too much towards the latter risks making oneself a mere post-holder, lacking imagination, flexibility and genuine personal ethical accountability. One can be alienated from one's work and one's official role either way – either by seeing oneself as detached from it or by seeing oneself as defined by it.[11] Thus – up to a point – a tension between vocational and institutional identities is intrinsic to professionalism. Also it is important to recognize that individuals do not need to be wholly coherent and univocal in the way they work. There is room for sharing this tension with clients and for using it creatively to keep more than one issue and perspective on the table. The health visitors in the Greenway et al. study, for example, self-consciously engaged in this kind of strategy – saying things like 'something I am supposed to discuss with you', 'another thing they tell me to ask about'. This use of an overtly hybrid professional identity overlaps with the second approach to balancing control and autonomy described above.

Living with power: a fundamental challenge for professionals

As we hope is clear throughout this book and is explicit in the last two sections, occupying a professional role has both social and personal dimensions. If professionals are interested in doing the right thing, they need to be able to understand and to be reflexive about these dimensions and the interactions between them. They need, for example, to be able to see the ways in which the immediate needs of their individual clients might sometimes be subordinated to the social goals that are built into their working agendas (the subject of the last-but-one section). They also need to be able to see that the ways in which their own personal values can either be put at risk by, or inflected through, the norms that are institutionally imposed on them (the subject of the last section). In both cases, we might worry about 'the personal' – whether that of the client or the professional – being effaced. As discussed in the last chapter, there seems to be a permanent risk of the uniqueness of the individual person getting lost in generalized norms and systems.

However, we can look at this same tension more constructively. We might, for example, embrace a model of integrity as including a consciousness of, and a continuous engagement with, these ubiquitous tensions. It is essential to understand that to occupy a professional role and be in relationship with a service user is necessarily to be in a different position than if one is acting purely as an individual agent in relation to someone else. Acting in a professional role cannot just mean confining oneself to whatever one is personally comfortable with and ignoring broader social complications. It requires attention to the social and political realities in which one is embedded. This applies above all to the overarching tension with which we began the chapter – the tension between professionals as 'powerful experts', on the one hand, and professionals as 'supporters or carers', on the other. Each individual professional needs to be ready to address this tension both over time, through collective processes of discussion and debate within their professional group, and moment by moment in their individual decisions and practices.

The social nature of professional roles means that individual practitioners may sometimes feel compromised by the identities that are 'thrust upon them', but it also means – and this is much easier to overlook – that these individual practitioners, however unassuming and humble they may be, automatically carry with them the authority and social power of the roles they occupy.[12] The business of professional surveillance, introduced in chapter 2 and arguably the most widely discussed concern about the power of professionals, can be used to illustrate this.

Surveillance (along with a number of related Foucauldian ideas) represents a familiar sociological theme in the analysis of professional work. It can be and has been applied to the example with which we began this chapter – that is, the work of health visitors in relation to mothers and families. At a superficial level, it refers to the kind of routine monitoring that health visitors and many other health and social care practitioners are charged with – for example, collecting data on well-being-related indices like weight or checking compliance with recommendations. To capture this, we can add the image of the professional as social police officer to the images that we mentioned at the start of the chapter, professionals as either social legislators or social servants. At a deeper level, however, the concept of surveillance illuminates the inherent links between professional knowledge and roles and the normative construction of subjectivity. The normative power of professionals runs very deep. The power of health visitors, for example, does not simply reside in the overt fact of them checking on and encouraging breastfeeding but on a whole complex of diffuse social processes. In particular, what lies behind their interactions with mothers of young babies is that the latter are subject to systems of authoritative expertise embodying norms of good and bad, right and wrong that do not only penetrate their homes but also their own self-consciousness. Mothers, in this instance, just as in the example of pregnancy and childbirth used in chapter 1, are brought face to face with powerful expectations of how they ought to be behaving. These are expectations which they are bound to take seriously, not least because they want to do their best for their babies, and expectations which either colonize their own thoughts or, even if they are inclined to resist them, exert normative pressure. Individual practitioners are thus not only powerful through their own immediate actions – which, like Saira, they might creatively moderate or modify – but also simply through being embedded in certain systems of thought and action. (In the breastfeeding case, for example, there is simply no need for the health visitor to say or do anything at all for this agenda to be present in the encounter with the mothers.)

The wide-ranging and deep-seated processes through which surveillance works pose a significant challenge for professional integrity. A health and social care practitioner cannot, or at least cannot straightforwardly, decide whether or not to be a social police officer. They can (so far as it is compatible with holding down their job) be very flexible about how thoroughly they collect data. They can try to be very flexible and tolerant in their attitudes to service users. In short, they can try to minimize the practices of surveillance in the superficial sense summarized above. However, they cannot detach themselves from the broader care system and deeper processes of power. They inevitably represent a socially powerful form of expertise and carry with them (however lightly) normative constructions of health and well-being. Even if the professional themselves might choose to dissociate themselves from dominant expectations in their field, they cannot reasonably expect their client or service user to recognize or attach any weight to such disassociation. This means that, to put it in crude terms, the dilemma for an individual professional is often not whether to be a social police officer but *how* to be a social police officer. There are burdens of association and of power that attach to professional roles. It might be nice for some practitioners to imagine that their 'hands are clean' and that their work stands outside of politics but ultimately this is just wishful thinking on their part. A more realistic (and more mature) stance involves recognizing that there is nothing of very much value that can be done without dirtying or even damaging one's hands and that the power of professionals can serve good as well as bad ends. Indeed, as we set out in the last chapter, having the power to do good is very close to the definition of professionalism as expertise-based social authority.

Conclusion

To exercise professionalism in the face of the continuous and sometimes major tensions and dilemmas that we have reviewed in this chapter is enormously exacting. It requires the

intellectual and ethical virtues and the emotional strengths
reviewed at the end of the previous chapter. It entails navigat-
ing through inherently intractable conflicts about purposes
and priorities and an indefinitely large number of more or less
visible, and more or less dramatic, ethical dilemmas about service design, individual comportment and social relationships.
But it entails more than this, including: a readiness to question
whether or not one's role allows one to exercise professionalism and whether and how one can best go about confronting
limitations; and a willingness and ability to acknowledge and
manage the tensions between one's vocational and institutional identities. Professionalism is not about conforming
to dominant official conceptions of one's role or good practice, but about the ability to understand, and work between,
competing conceptions. An understanding of the dilemmatic
nature of professionalism means not being focused on 'what
works' at the expense of a readiness to engage in debates about
what could count as working from case to case. In this chapter,
we have considered some of the dilemmas facing practitioners aiming to exercise professionalism. However, as set out
in the account of professionalism offered in chapter 4, this is
only half of the story. Professionalism can only be practised at
the individual level if the social institutions that make professionalism possible are in place. Establishing and maintaining
these institutions also gives rise to dilemmas and this is the
subject of the following chapter.

CHAPTER SIX

Supporting Professionalism

Although professionalism depends upon personal accomplishment it is, first and foremost, a social accomplishment. This is both because it depends upon social coordination (in that respect, it is like orchestral music, which includes but transcends the contributions of individual instrumentalists) and because, unless the enabling conditions are firmly in place, it is either impossible or extremely difficult to operate as an individual professional (as if, for example, the members of an orchestra had no instruments, or too few instruments, or no opportunities to rehearse). In this chapter, we will explore some general questions about the social conditions of professionalism – what kinds of conditions need to be in place and what are the challenges and choices involved in creating and maintaining these conditions? This chapter thus continues the discussion of tensions and dilemmas started in the previous chapter, but it shifts the focus to those agencies and agents who have roles in and responsibilities for shaping and supporting professional work. It is worth noting from the start that successes and failures of professionalism often belong just as much to this 'arm's length' group of people as they do to individual practitioners 'on the ground'. When we think about ethics in professional life, for example, we would be wrong to focus exclusively on the latter. Ethical issues arise in relation to the construction and support of professional roles and not only in relation to their enactment.

Here, we have a number of different kinds of agents in mind – some of whom have a relatively direct effect on professional roles and the possibilities of professionalism and some who have a more indirect effect. In the former category, we would include managers and employers, and lying behind them, but in a broadly comparable position, various kinds of policy makers and regulators. In the latter category, we are thinking primarily of those with a formal or informal education role. We also have in mind those people who work for, or play a significant role in the structures of, professional bodies, and these can fall into both categories (depending on the precise remit or section of the body in question). This reference to professional bodies allows us to stress at the outset that there is no clear separation between the categories of professionals and managers, or between those 'on the ground' and those at 'arm's length' from practice. One of the traditional planks of professionalism is, of course, the notion that professionals are to some degree self-governing (or, in other words, have collective autonomy) and, although the reality of this varies, it is important to keep this in mind as we proceed. In what follows, we will return to some of the issues and tensions we have already discussed but look at them through a different frame.

Managing professionals – accountability as audit

As we have explored in previous chapters, there has been a rise in certain kinds of control over the work of health and social care professionals. This is manifest in the use of targets, incentives and performance management systems in combination with the growth of evidence-based forms of governance, often accompanied by institutional rules, protocols or prescribed toolkits, and resource sets (for example, institutional drug formularies). Taken as a whole these shifts mark the ascendancy and dominance of a particular, and particularly narrow, notion of professional accountability – according to which practitioners have not only to continually demonstrate what they are doing in concrete (preferably measurable) terms but have also thereby to demonstrate that they are doing whatever is institutionally preferred or even dictated. This is a model of accountability that is defined around 'audit' and the increasing subsumption of individual judgement by institutional judgement. The rise of this narrow version of institutional accountability has occurred in parallel with, and is partly informed by, substantial pressures for cost containment and this tendency has been described by some as the triumph of 'accounting logic' in professional work.[1] This is not just because of the concern over monies per se but, more fundamentally, because of the drive to make more and more things – including the substantive content of professional work – auditable, that is, both visible to managers and calculable by them.

This broad shift towards an audit conception of accountability has been the cause of extensive controversy. Professionals often report feeling frustrated and undermined by it and complain about its effects on their role and the quality of their work. It has also been subjected to substantial critique by both academic and popular commentators. We are very sympathetic to these critiques and, as we will go on to discuss below, it is arguable that some implementations of this change have been responsible for very profound damage to the substance of professional work and thus to clients and service users. However, before following this critical line, it is important to recognize that there are often good intentions, and some good arguments, behind aspects of this shift. Problems arise with the model when particular elements are combined together in particular ways – the elements are certainly not all bad in themselves.

There are obviously very good arguments for trying to limit both poor practice and wasted resources. Everyone, not least, patients or service users, stands to benefit from this. If a doctor has been routinely using a treatment for a purpose for which, according to all the evidence, it is ineffective (or worse), then that may not only amount to a substantial waste of resources (which, of course, could do some good elsewhere) but may also result in significant harm to the patient. If we imagine that there are more effective (and perhaps also less expensive) treatments available, we could reasonably view the continuation of this poor practice as a case of negligence at the system level. Why, we would ask – and we can imagine the family of the patient concerned asking – has this been allowed to continue? Why hasn't someone done something about it? Under these circumstances, it would seem reasonable to institute relevant guidelines and treatment protocols and formal and informal systems of 'steering' the doctor in a more cost-effective direction. We would also expect someone who wanted to continue with unorthodox and questionable treatment choices to face the scrutiny and challenge of professional colleagues and – unless the individual concerned was able to justify themselves despite the prevailing consensus about normal good practice – to be subjected to constraints or even sanctions. In this case, the practicalities and the logic of audit and performance review seem to fit reasonably well.

The 'steering' of professionals (rather than allowing them to wholly steer themselves) may also be justified when some degree of social coordination serves an important collective end. For example, given the very serious worries that exist about the over-prescribing of antibiotics (specifically, the public health dangers of these becoming ineffective through the unintended increase in population resistance to them), some collective action seems necessary. There may be no compelling reason why any particular individual practitioner, considered in isolation, should moderate their use of antibiotics, but there is a compelling reason for every individual practitioner to do so when the whole picture is taken into account. Under these circumstances, the routine audit of practice and the encouragement of compliance with guidelines (with something like the use of targets and rewards as a mechanism) can make sense.

There is, however, a tendency to extend this same logic, and the same mechanisms, to other cases where the fit can be less clear-cut. Although the prescribing model is quite a good analogue for many interventions, it is not always so – often the interventions concerned are fuzzier and the nature of the evidence is much more contested. In other words, there is often much more scope for legitimate professional disagreement (there is, of course, often scope for disagreement in prescribing decisions, too). Also, in many instances, it is much less easy to separate out the 'active ingredient' in an intervention and thereby to differentiate 'professional style' from intervention 'substance'. For example, in 'talking' or broader social interventions, the way practitioners operate – their characters and interpersonal or political approaches – determines their effectiveness and is something that is much less readily analysed into intervention components and generalized about.

There are also problems attached to extending an approach that is motivated by a desire to avoid the harms of poor practice, or to manage collective risks, to the promotion of positive ends. Although there is no clear analytical separation between these two things, there are often different considerations and emphases that need to be taken seriously. It might be worth drawing a very loose parallel here for illustrative purposes: imagine we are trying to regulate the work that goes on in a restaurant kitchen. We might begin with health and safety concerns in mind. We could establish some fairly firm rules about, for example, the storage of food and the cleaning of surfaces and equipment. We might also institute a systematic model for checking that rules are being complied with, and for recording and reviewing the checks, along with a system of incentives and disincentives to help motivate the relevant staff to adhere to the rules. Suppose all that seems to work very well and it not only allows us to reduce the number of harmful incidents but to demonstrate that fact to stakeholders and customers. Bolstered by our success, we decide to extend the model to everything that happens in the kitchen. In future, chefs will be required to follow pre-set rules and to systematically demonstrate that they are doing so as they proceed. We then set about defining menus, recipes, protocols and recording procedures for every task involved. It is easy to see that this model might work reasonably well for a fast-food restaurant producing standard meals, but it is not one that anyone who aspired to be a good cook or chef could remotely accept. Indeed, it might be said that it is one in which cooking – and everything that makes it creative, meaningful or worthwhile – has effectively been abolished. For a restaurant that aspires to quality, it makes no sense to extend a model developed to manage safety to these other more substantive areas. It would make just as much sense to say that, having made a successful lamb stew, we should apply exactly the same cooking procedures to making a chocolate cake – to ensure that it too is successful.

Of course, many of the relevant examples in health and social care, including the examples discussed earlier in the book, are in a middle ground. There are aspects of them that are analogous to poor or risky treatment choices and there are aspects of them that are more like undermining the creative scope of an aspiring chef and thus the possibility of quality provision. Health visitors (or GPs) who are expected to structure some of their work around public health targets, or social workers who are expected to deliver on equivalent targets, are being encouraged to meet important collective ends, but they can also feel they are thereby being denied the creative licence to deal responsively and imaginatively with the different individuals and circumstances they encounter. In all of these cases, it is necessary to take a thoughtful, fine-grained and context-sensitive approach to determining the right balance. This is the core dilemma for managers and employing institutions – how, in principle and in practice, to combine and balance the advantages and disadvantages of what we might call, in shorthand, 'enforcement' and 'encouragement'. (As we will underline and explore shortly, managers and employers are not the only relevant agents here, and indeed they are themselves subject to much of the same audit and accounting logic and mechanisms that we are considering.)

It is impossible to over-stress the importance of this dilemma. Not only the quality but even the very possibility of professionalism depends upon addressing it conscientiously, sensitively and rigorously. Just as in the kitchen example, the risk is that something that starts off as a plausible approach to doing one thing (the prevention of dangerous or otherwise bad practice) ends up doing something very different (the abolition of best practice). The reason that the conditions for professionalism are under threat if the collective response to this dilemma is mishandled was indicated in chapter 4. Professionalism, as we are advocating it, represents a form of expertise-based social authority and influence. If there is insufficient 'elbow room' for practitioners to use their hard-won experience, know-how, judgement and discretion to help shape their own working conditions and practices, they will all be in the same position as aspiring cooks who are expected to turn out standard – and often neither tasty nor nutritious – fast-food meals. The potentially negative effects of 'overdoing' a narrow audit-based approach to accountability are manifold but include: breeding resentment and demotivation (even when – or because – practitioners are directed to do what they would do in any case); reducing flexibility of provision and thereby scope for personalization that reflects individual or context variables; encouraging 'working to targets', making targets the priority, rather than attempting to reflect and act upon all relevant needs and making service users the priority; and in some cases generating a tendency on the part of practitioners to 'game the system' or even engage in distortion or fraud so as to 'perform' adequately according to measures, rather than face up to the much more troubling business of acknowledging potential service limitations or challenges.

Fortunately – as noted above – there is a spectrum between enforcement and encouragement; there are some alternatives to the most coercive forms of professional control and ways of moderating and complementing them. Within institutions and teams, good practice is often underpinned, shared and enhanced by more dispersed processes – formal and informal workplace learning, firmly established values and principles (embedded in practices and working cultures and norms) that manifest an aspiration to serve a client group, and official and unofficial leadership which comes in many different shapes and sizes and can sometimes be subtle and gentle (or high-energy and infectious), rather than rigidly prescriptive. Indeed the full repertoire of management encompasses these forms of leadership including values-based climate-setting and professional example; and it should not be forgotten that one's managers are sometimes also one's professional colleagues who are, or have recently been, in a similar boat and may well have both empathy about, and insight into, the demands of professional work. It is a mistake to assume there is anything inherently narrow (and thereby destructive) about management.

In the second part of the chapter, we will consider some of the less prescriptive and more informal and cultural forms of professional leadership and influence – particularly the example of educational influence – and some of the dilemmas associated with them. But before moving on, we should acknowledge there is not only widespread scepticism within health and social care about the corrosive effects of accounting logic and managerialism, there is also scepticism about how far it is possible to transcend this narrow model and to 're-balance' approaches to the management and leadership of professionals. This is because there are other layers of agencies and agents, and broader socio-economic processes behind both front-line and institutional managers. These other layers and processes, in turn, compromise managers' capacity to be creative themselves – to respond imaginatively to the needs of their services and to use more flexible and constructive models of accountability. The key problem is not merely that the professionals have increasingly been narrowly managed but also that their managers have increasingly been narrowly managed.

Indeed, it is arguable that the principal locus for the logic and mechanism of performance management and accounting logic is the institution rather than the individual practitioner. Whole institutions and services are given targets and sets of incentives/disincentives, and it is typically these same pressures and measures that are then 'relayed' through the service to the practitioners. Policy makers and senior service leaders thus have a fundamental role in, and responsibility for, setting the conditions for professional work and for the possibility and 'health' of professionalism. Once again, some of the rationale for this institutional management is constructive, but there is the same risk and tendency for it to be over-extended in ways that are destructive rather than productive. That is to say, it clearly makes sense for institutions to be accountable for their work, and it can certainly be helpful for them to have some framework of expectations and guidance about their purpose. However, if this logic is operationalized too narrowly and rigidly, it is liable to create as much damage as benefit. Of course, as noted elsewhere, some of this 'collateral damage' is also a product of pressures for cost containment which either accompany or, very often, are built into the targets and incentive structures deployed. In so far as this whole process is damaging, it is difficult to disentangle the extent to which the distorting effects on professionalism come from attempts to specify standards and practices or from the allied – and substantial – push towards cost containment and service efficiency.

It is key to the success of this approach to institutional management (and the local management of professionals) that it rests on premises which have plausibility and some intellectual and ethical legitimacy. To return to where this section started, it is, of course, important to use resources responsibly, to avoid waste and to seek to eliminate poor practice and promote good practice. It makes sense for everyone within an institution to be seen to do a 'good job', and institutional and professional targets can harness the loyalty of staff at all levels to do their best to meet institutional performance targets so as to protect their own service and the budget that makes their work possible. There is no need to assume that anyone is setting out to wreck things. Quite the contrary. However, just as we need to study side effects of practice interventions, we need to be alive, and pay close attention, to the serious side effects of policy interventions.

Learning and leading – enabling intelligent accountability

Institutions and individuals do need to be accountable for their practices and their successes and failures. But, at the same time, it is important not to stifle the flexibility, creativity or motivation of practitioners, and it is important that systems of accountability do not become part of the problem rather than the solution. These dilemmas of professional accountability are not easily resolved. But any serious attempt at a resolution will include education as a crucial ingredient. Here we are referring to education at every level and of every kind, not just the pre-service preparation of practitioners, but the broader and more diffuse forms of practical and theoretical learning that are available in the contexts of work and policy-making. This is, of course, only to repeat one of the core tenets of conventional accounts of professionalism. Professions rest upon the idea of expertise and of suitable learning and assessment trajectories for the cultivation and practice of expertise.

An example

Lauren is a new GP and she is worried about reconciling her own ideas about good practice with the various expectations in her workplace. This is partly a concern about the framework of targets and measures that she is being expected to follow, but it extends more broadly. There are occasions when she feels that targets get in the way of the consultation with the individual patient; and there are also demands from patients and from other colleagues that sometimes seem to pull in conflicting directions. Some of these tensions are fairly minor (for example, her computer reminds her that she should be measuring someone's blood pressure to comply with the practice's targets at a time when she is involved in a very intense exchange with the patient about something important and unrelated), but others seem potentially more worrying to her. For example, she is being encouraged to keep the blood glucose level of her patients between certain levels, but she is aware of contrary evidence that suggests that these limits may not be appropriate for some of her elderly patients. In addition, she has built up a good working relationship with a nurse practitioner who is a specialist in supporting diabetes patients and who is sceptical about the targets and also stresses the importance of working in partnership with patients so as to agree aims and negotiate treatment regimes that are realistic for, and 'owned by', them. This broad person-centred approach seems right to Lauren and echoes what she learned in medical school. On the other hand, she is anxious that her patients get the best clinical treatment and she is uncomfortable about them being given too much scope to 'drift away' from what is clinically demanded. Finally, Lauren is unsure about how much to share her uncertainties with the patients directly – should she be explaining about the official targets or sharing her own dilemmas with patients, or are both of these things unfair and unkind and simply compounding the concerns of patients who come, at least sometimes, for reassuring and relatively clear advice, and not to share her professional burdens? Lauren takes her unease to Angela, a senior colleague in the practice who is acting as her mentor. Angela can see that Lauren is troubled. She can see that Lauren wants to do a good job and to be seen as a competent and effective member of the practice. Lauren, she recognizes, doesn't want to be demanding or disruptive, but she does want to raise questions about how to operate in a complex environment.[2]

Our interest here is not to directly debate what Angela should say or do, but simply to identify this mentoring relationship as one significant point in a web of educational processes. Perhaps it is first worth noting that to position Angela as an 'educator' in this way is not at all fanciful. Most professional organizations (including, in this case, for example, the General Medical Council in the United Kingdom and the Australian Medical Association) list education, including the training and mentoring of colleagues, as an official requirement of professional roles. The line that Angela takes is not only likely to have a significant influence over Lauren's future practice orientation but it may also strongly inform her sense of professionalism. For example, is she encouraged and enabled to be reflective about the worries that she has and to air them and debate them with colleagues, or is this kind of reflexivity more or less subtly 'dampened down' with a heavy dose of pragmatism or even cynicism? The tone and substance of the dialogue with Angela could form a crucial moment in Lauren's professional trajectory. Clearly, it is not simply a question of *what* is said but *how* things are said. Furthermore, this interaction will be nested inside Lauren's perception of Angela's character and own conduct. Is Angela, let us say, someone who seems to embody a thoughtful and responsible approach to her role? Is she ready to be reflective herself? Can she be self-critical and admit her own limitations and uncertainties, as well as offering supportive advice?

The education of health and social care professionals involves developing and supporting a broad range of different kinds of knowledge (as discussed in chapter 4). This includes some quite narrow competences – knowledge of specific technical skills or knowledge of specific facts of law, for example. But it also encompasses developing an understanding of the broader (and contested) principles and purposes that provide the rationale for professional work, and the chance to practise capabilities in diverse (and unpredictable) settings in which narrow competences are necessary but insufficient. It also includes character development and the encouragement and support of the ethical and intellectual virtues that underpin both the motivation and the discriminating power of the professional mindset. Professional education is thus an incredibly complex and long-term undertaking. Different settings, practices and occasions will help foster or sustain different facets of the necessary expertise. Some academic settings, such as seminars in pre-service courses, may provide an insight into theoretical underpinnings or some of the ethical and political contests that frame debates about purposes and priorities. These same seminars may, however, neglect some of the practical contingencies of workplace organization.[3] The reverse is true in other settings. In an ideal world, these different learning experiences will be complementary to one another and will overlap enough for the learner to be able to see the connections between different facets of expertise and not to see them as located in insulated and disconnected pockets.

Of course, the encounter described above does not take place in a formal educational setting. There will not be time to tease out all of the possible complications and interpretations. To some extent, both parties will be conscious of the need to get on with their jobs and to find practical ways of working rather than getting bogged down in an open-ended exploration of possibilities. Nonetheless, there is scope for Angela to draw on her own education and professional development, and to make the experience more or less continuous with the experiences and lessons Lauren encountered in her formal training. One of the challenges facing many professionals is the disjunction between the philosophies espoused in training contexts and the pragmatics of coping day to day. Lauren has been taught about, and is motivated by, the idea of person-centredness and she is now facing the challenge of trying to make this idea work under pressure with conflicting instincts about what it involves. Lauren is also encountering the demands of accountability in a heightened way. She wishes to be a loyal and effective employee, but she is experiencing multiple accountabilities first-hand, including accountabilities to her patients, her colleagues, her profession and to herself and her own sense of proper conduct. The issue of targets, and the accompanying accountability to her employers and official policies, is only one aspect of this situation. This example reminds us (as discussed in chapter 5) that there are innumerable dilemmas and tensions that professionals face that are much broader than and 'pre-exist' concerns about audit and performance measurement.

There are many things that Angela might usefully do or say in response. There is no single right response at that moment (given there will be future opportunities also), and exactly what is effective will depend upon many things, including her own character and personal style, and her developing relationship with Lauren. But some things that might be helpful include: (1) showing a recognition of the uncertainties Lauren is facing and their legitimacy; (2) discussing the official basis of the practice's policies and guidelines – clarifying the 'facts' – and her own perception of them and the existing scope for flexibility built into them; (3) acknowledging the inherent dilemmas in balancing different considerations – both evidence-related and value-related – and (if true) her own feelings of inadequacy, on occasions, with resolving competing conceptions of what is for the best; (4) suggesting that they get together with the specialist nurse practitioner in the area (and possibly other colleagues) to review their practice generally and jointly consider some individual patient histories to see if they can collectively explore what can and should be done in specific cases – both with regard to treatment targets and management but also in terms of shared decision-making and supporting patient self-management; and (5) exploring what broader support might be available to them (through external training or web materials, etc.) to take the discussion forward – including drawing on the voice of 'expert patients' and patient organizations as well as professional bodies or health service improvement agencies.

Some combination of responses along these lines have the potential to make Lauren feel – rightly – that her feelings and questions are positively contributing to the support of professionalism, rather than simply being an unwelcome 'drain' on colleagues' valuable time. These responses would also serve to exemplify the importance of working respectfully across professional boundaries, as well as with patients, and the value of working and developing practice collectively.

This example illustrates, in microcosm, the routine opportunities for learning, and enabling learning, in practice contexts. Of course, the options open to Angela and Lauren, and how easy it feels for them to think in terms such as mentorship or learning, or to foster further group learning, will depend upon the culture of their workplace and the wider system. In this respect, what can be said about education is similar to what was said about audit in the previous section. A broader culture of learning can reinforce individual learning efforts just as an institutional culture of compliance can reinforce a compliance mindset at an individual level. As we emphasized earlier, there can sometimes be an important role for audit and compliance. But, and this is what we are hoping to underline here, both knowing where that place is and being aware of its boundaries ensures that practice takes place within a learning culture and ideally within a 'learning organization'.[4] The literature on workplace learning problematizes a simple model of learning as acquisition based on planned learning interventions, emphasizing instead the broader contextual and unplanned factors that make learning more or less possible and create the conditions for either more 'expansive' or more 'restrictive' learning environments.[5] Education is sometimes thought of as an 'easy' or 'soft' area – the domain of 'keeping up to date' with evidence or skills, and of 'personal development' and so forth. However, we suggest that, properly understood, education also involves individuals and groups confronting the very hard – technically, emotionally and ethically hard – questions about organizing and providing care and, not least, of taking responsibility for these things.

Both Lauren and Angela are taking responsibility. They are not just minimally filling a role but helping to shape and develop the role they fill. They take their personal accountability for what they are doing seriously and personal accountability here means something much richer and broader than accountability in the audit sense. It is broader because it does not focus on a few performance indicators but includes a much more extensive – indeed, indefinitely large – set of considerations. It is richer because it demands more than a bureaucratic performance but involves drawing upon their intellectual, emotional and social resources. Another way of describing this kind of responsibility, and the interaction between Lauren and Angela, is to talk in terms of 'leadership'. Lauren and Angela (and the specialist nurse practitioner mentioned in the scenario) could be said to be exercising leadership. We will say a little more about this reading before returning to the idea of accountability.

Leadership is a huge and important subject which we can only touch upon here. There are many different taxonomies of leadership approaches or 'styles' and many guides to, and resources on, leadership.[6] However, in simple terms, leadership is the exercise of social influence within a team or organization so as to help colleagues articulate and realize the purposes of the team or organization. It is important to stress that, at least according to definitions and models that have widespread influence in health and social care (and many other sectors too), leadership is not the same as management and does not relate to particular positions in organizational hierarchies. Leadership can be exercised in teams that are 'flat' as well as within hierarchical structures, and by any individual from any position – this idea is sometimes referred to as 'shared leadership' or 'distributed leadership'.[7] What matters is whether individuals have the dispositions and capabilities to influence their colleagues, rather than who or what they

are. Although some people will have more scope for exercising leadership than others, everyone has some scope. Those
who occupy officially designated leadership positions face particular challenges and have specific responsibilities. It falls
to them to be directly accountable for providing supportive
working conditions, for ensuring educational and training
opportunities and for holding colleagues to account for lapses
or for poor performance more broadly. Furthermore – as we
outlined in chapter 3 – they often have to do this under heavy
resource constraints and in institutional settings that are
far from ideal. This is not an obvious recipe for popularity.
However, it is arguably a duty for all would-be professionals to
recognize this fact and to share, and thereby lessen, some of
this leadership burden as far as they feel able.

This conception of leadership (as organizational influence)
is very closely related to the notion of professionalism we have
been discussing throughout the book. It is just one expression
of what should be expected from, and needs supporting in,
professionalism. It is also very closely related to the theme of
learning that we have used to organize this section. This is
both because leadership involves creating learning opportunities for others and also because it is not feasible for someone to
be an effective leader if they are not themselves in the habit of
listening and learning.

One of the reasons that the health and social care professions
have embraced the language of leadership (and established all
kinds of related educational and policy interventions to support
leadership as an intrinsic part of professionalism) is because it
enables them to reassert the importance of professional influence and authority in a climate in which there has been a risk
of bureaucratic authority dominating. The distinction between
leadership and management, in the narrow managerialist
sense, is just one example of the tension between occupational
and organizational professionalism. Of course, as noted above,
there are broader conceptions of management that can incorporate the idea of leadership and complement audit models with

a vision or organizational purpose, and broader conceptions of accountability and evaluation. The challenge is how to hold these two emphases together because there will be ongoing conflicts between bureaucratic constructions of accountability and the lived experience of personal accountability.

Working contexts that are able to combine rich learning and leadership environments make possible more intelligent forms of accountability[8] that recognize both the need for institutional accountability systems and the importance of 'owned' accountability for individual and groups of professionals. In broad terms, what we are calling intelligent accountability means not only or not necessarily saying to professionals 'your targets are a, b and c', but rather saying 'you are expected to deliver good quality care and service bearing in mind x aims, y objectives and z principles and we require you to demonstrate how you are interpreting and delivering on x, y and z and how you are evaluating your practices and outcomes.' In practice, this may well include recourse to some standardized measures, but it will also encourage innovation and creativity in working practices and in models of evaluation. Although intelligent accountability of this sort is in some respects more challenging at an organizational level, it has the potential to harness much more effectively the full epistemic and ethical resources of all staff to promote productive professional dialogue, to foster local flexibility and responsiveness and thereby to generate substantial system-wide benefits.

The idea of intelligent accountability echoes Donald Schön's celebrated account of valuable professional practice in which he stresses the importance of 'flexible procedures', 'differentiated responses' and 'decentralised responsibility for judgement and action' as conditions for both reflective practice and wider organizational learning.[9] There are also strong parallels between the conditions needed for intelligent accountability and those needed for creating expansive learning environments.[10] The models of accountability and professional development employed by organizations send very powerful messages about what does and does not matter. If we want to support professionalism, we need to pay very careful attention to these message systems.

Conclusion

For health and social care practitioners to have the opportunity to exercise professionalism, the right social and organizational building blocks need to be put in place. This means that the fundamental responsibility for professionalism in these domains rests with policy makers, institutional managers and those in formal and informal leadership positions within professional groups. Unless these agents effectively address the challenges they face, it is simply unreasonable to expect very much from individuals on the ground. We might expect individuals to put in effort and to do their best to benefit rather than harm service users, but the quantity and quality of their contribution will be very heavily circumscribed. When social resources are lacking, the situation is exactly analogous to the absence of physical resources. Surgeons can do so much more if they have operating facilities and equipment than if they do not. Professionalism more generally depends upon key pieces of social equipment. For example, if we think back to Helen, the paediatric oncology outreach nurse specialist discussed in chapter 4, her ability to do the job is determined by many things, including: her voice and experience being 'licensed' and heard in a range of settings; effective networks of communication and care coordination; and a fair degree of flexibility and responsiveness in relation to working schedules and tasks. Without these things, no amount of effort could get the job done.

The social organization of professionalism is by no means easy. It involves tackling very difficult balancing acts and dilemmas. There is obviously a need for some rules and regulations. There is a place for guidelines and targets of various kinds. But the very nature of professionalism means that these can only be one part of the mix. As we have tried to show in this chapter, there is a constant need to balance enforcement and encouragement, to support both 'top-down' and 'bottom-up' leadership, and to create environments which are conducive to professional learning. Clearly, accountability has to run through all levels of the system. When there are shortfalls in professional standards or ethics, we need to be at least as ready to examine the failures of those who have the most power within the system as we are to call to account those operating on the ground.

In order to effectively support professionalism, we obviously need some broad notion of what professionalism is and entails. The account we have offered here and in the previous two chapters of a form of professionalism that is compatible with contemporary social and working conditions has, we hope, helped to fill out such a notion. We have highlighted the 'dilemmatic' nature of professionalism in health and social care – that is, the fact that professionalism involves the continuous negotiation of value tensions and practical judgements. More specifically, we have stressed that the more collaborative models of professionalism required in a social context that is more sceptical about authority demand careful and responsive social negotiation and relational as well as technical forms of expertise. Such professionals will need to be 'critically reflexive'. They will need to be ready to acknowledge the potential weaknesses as well as the strengths of the lines they take. They will need to be comfortable in engaging with the challenges and doubts of others, and they will need to be supported in acknowledging and managing their own self-doubts. They will have the capacity to work at a 'human level' – that is, to draw on their own personal resources and to connect with the experiences and perspectives of others. They will be ready to share and demystify their expertise and they will take it for granted both that they have accountabilities towards the communities they work with (as well as their professional organization or the state) and that they have a civic role in using their expertise to contribute at least to some degree to public life. In short, such professionals are likely to be both more 'human' and more democratic in spirit.

CHAPTER SEVEN

Professional Identities

In this final chapter, we want to summarize the key ideas and implications of the book by asking some questions about professionalism from the standpoint of the individual practitioner. This involves a change of emphasis from the discussion in the previous chapter of the social coordination and support of professionalism. There, we were focused on what is needed to 'orchestrate' professionalism; here, we will be thinking more about the position of individual players – each of whom will, of course, have their own biographies, identities, concerns, motivations and perspectives. For that very reason, it is impossible for us to cover the myriad number of potentially relevant issues in a single chapter. Rather, we will continue to present our argument in a relatively general, impersonal and theoretical fashion. However, we hope that the questions we ask will be of relevance to many individuals and we would encourage readers to 'personalize' these for themselves and, ideally, to consider their own possible responses.

The chapter – like the book as a whole – might, we hope, encourage a certain kind of expansive reflective practice. At the most basic, each of us can ask the book's organizing questions of ourselves: Is professionalism possible for me and, if so, how far is it desirable? Those people who are still coming to terms with fulfilling a professional role may find it worthwhile to explore their own uncertainties and to recognize that such uncertainties often reflect the complexity of the territory rather than anything about themselves personally. Those who are more experienced may find it helpful to reflect on what is entailed by the challenge of professionalism in order to better support others including their present and future colleagues. For, we would suggest, exercising professionalism is in effect being a custodian of a certain kind of role. In other words, it is not only about trying to perform one's role well, but it is also about trying to understand the social formation of, and pressures on, occupational roles and about trying to develop and 'pass on' to others – through example, education or social action – whatever it is that makes one's work valuable.

Am I a professional? Am I professional?

Not everyone identifies with the category of profession or professionalism. This includes many people who happily fill what others might readily label as professional roles. Indeed, some of these people would wish to positively distance themselves from such labels (we know this because we have asked a lot of people, including ourselves). This is partly because, as we discussed in chapter 2, these terms carry multiple connotations and 'stretch' in many directions – they suggest different things to different people. It is also because these terms are inherently contested and 'Janus-faced' – they face in the direction of ideals, like public service and altruism, and they face in the direction of the social distance, hierarchy and exclusion associated with the status connotations of professionalism.

Many people who work in health and social care are primarily motivated by the substance of the work they do – both the instrumental benefits to others and the intrinsic meaningfulness of the contribution – rather than the way their role is socially defined. More specifically, they may want to resist the idea that they are somehow 'special' and worry that their official role, and the assumptions and practices that go along with it, separate them off from the people they work with. In short, they may fill a professional role but wish to dissociate themselves from 'brand professional'. This worry is especially common for practitioners who have a strong sense that their role depends on working collaboratively and closely with individuals and communities, for example, those who are interested in helping to facilitate and support community development initiatives. In some cases the personal identities of individuals may also make the assertion of a professional identity uncomfortable. For example, in areas where the dominant images of professionals are those of white middle-class men, and where certain conventions of dress, comportment and conduct dominate, people from other, diverse backgrounds and with different personal styles, histories and imagined futures may feel justified in pushing not only against these dominant images and norms but also against the very language of professionalism that seems to adhere to them.

Similarly, individuals can seek to do their job well, to strive to meet high standards and to embody what they believe to be the right qualities without invoking the idea that they are 'being professional'. They may accept this phrase as a common shorthand for their stance whilst personally preferring to use different descriptions. In other words, some practitioners might choose to give a 'Yes, but . . .' answer to the two questions in this section title. We are perfectly content for such people to read the rest of this chapter on professional identities with a different label in mind – 'practice identities', 'working identities', 'role identities' or some such. Likewise, they may have in mind other ways of emphasizing the standards or quality of their work practices and motivations than talking in terms of professionalism. However, before continuing, we should note that there is a certain 'objective' aspect to these matters that transcends individuals' self-identities. In this respect, being a professional is just like being a 'qualified driver'. If you want to be allowed to drive down the country's roads, you need to be prepared to fulfil some social requirements and pass certain tests. This then gives you certain entitlements and privileges and a corresponding set of responsibilities. If you want to be able to drive heavy goods vehicles or other specialist machinery, there are further hoops to jump through and extra entitlements and responsibilities. Someone is a qualified

driver, in this kind of sense, irrespective of whether they identify with the label or see it as a central or marginal part of their
personal identity. This is certainly the case for someone who
then actually accepts and works in a job as a driver. If such
a person were to deny their 'driver identity', we would wish
to examine their rationale quite carefully and might even be
aware, in some cases, of the possibility of self-deception.

Our focus is on people who are in socially sanctioned roles
that, in principle, involve them using their 'licensed' knowledge, capabilities and accumulated experience to work and
exercise influence in a certain practice domain – what we have
summarized as the use of expertise-based social authority.
We are interested in what is needed for such influence to be
deployed and exercised well. This, in essence, is what we mean
by professionalism.

Can my expertise be used for good?

Critiques of professions are not a marginal phenomenon.
They have become common currency. Reflective practitioners are liable to be conscious of these critiques, for example,
that professional ideology is a means of gaining social rewards,
and it is increasingly difficult to adopt a professional role on
the assumption that this is a wholly benign or innocent activity. Expertise can be used to dominate others. More generally,
authoritative systems of knowledge help to define who or what
is normal, natural, socially acceptable and so on, and this
implicates professionals in systems of social classification and
control. More prosaically, professionals are often gatekeepers
to resources and services that help determine, and so sometimes restrict, other people's access to goods and opportunities.
Individual professionals may often feel relatively powerless,
and there are sometimes good reasons for this, but this does
not mean that they are not also relatively powerful in relation to
service users. In particular, they (often unwittingly) channel
the huge organizational and discursive power of the systems

for which they work. These factors help explain why, as we have just rehearsed, for some people, a professional identity is a 'spoiled' identity.[1] As we have discussed in several places, concerns about the social power of professionals have been used to justify reforms that have attempted to circumscribe the power of professionals from both 'above' and 'below'. Such reforms may help to make practitioners sensitive to the dangers of too much licence, but at the same time they can also prevent them from supporting other people creatively and effectively.

This possibility of frustration reminds us not to lose sight of the fact that professionals can do good as well as harm, and not to over-stress the costs and risks of professional roles. It is a sign of maturity to recognize that most things are neither 'all bad' nor 'all good'. (In fact, the very few serious candidates for being wholly one or the other are abstractions and not socially embedded phenomena.) A feeling of ambivalence about the value of one's work is arguably a healthy sign rather than a worrying one. As we set out to help, care for, or otherwise support other individuals or groups, it would be worrying if we did not have some sense of the risks of so doing. On the other hand, if we were to continuously hold back from doing anything for fear of doing the wrong thing, directly or indirectly, we would be in danger of a kind of ethical paralysis that is difficult to justify. This is reasonably clear from the kind of emergency situation described in the opening of this book: if someone collapses in a public place and you have some relevant (first-aid or clinical) expertise – even if you have no legal duty – there is a reasonable moral expectation that you will do what you can to help. Things are even more clear-cut if you have accepted a role that formally carries an ethical obligation to care for others. As we discussed in chapter 4, the point of having knowledge is that it enables you to do some good. Our knowledge, our insight, our relevant experience can be underused as well as overused.

The challenge, then, is to find ways of using the various kinds of expertise, and the social licences and obligations we have, for good and at the same time to be critically reflexive about the things we do and the things we are implicated in. As we shall see in the subsequent sections, there are a number of demanding challenges facing practitioners who are ready to embrace ambivalence and critical reflection as well as their positive commitments to make a difference. But this is no more than is routinely entailed by life – especially life in a more questioning and sceptical era. We expect those people who drive ambulances to be very aware of the risks of the road and those who organize ambulance services to be mindful of the wider environmental burdens of ambulance use (for example, by limiting overall carbon emissions where possible). The same balancing acts apply to everyone else in health and social care.

How can I work with others respectfully?

Increasingly, the norm is to see the exercise of professionalism as something that is done *with* people rather than done *to* them. This expectation applies both to the development of strengthened and mutually respectful inter-professional partnerships and to less distant or hierarchical professional–client relationships, although here we will concentrate on the latter. Some of the language of 'new professionalism' – ideas like partnership or person-centredness – is designed to indicate and underpin this shift. A range of agendas is served by this new emphasis. For example, working collaboratively is often defended on the grounds of cost-effectiveness. It is argued that, rather than wasting resources by trying to get people to do things they could resist, it makes more sense to work with them to steer a course. But the fundamental ethical driver behind these changes is the recognition that people – whether 'professionals' or 'clients' – are equally important and equally deserving of respect. This important insight is sometimes condensed into the notion that professional–client relationships (like inter-professional relationships) have become, or need to become, 'more equal'. This may be a useful signpost, but it provides few clues as to what this entails in practice. We would suggest that, at the very least, it means thinking in terms of properly harnessing one's own 'person' and 'humanity' in one's professional role (which we will come back to in the next section), and thinking about the nature of relevant expertise in flexible and imaginative ways.

The kinds of expertise we are pointing to here extend well beyond both technical expertise and what are sometimes referred to as 'communication skills'. They are more fundamental forms of 'relational' or 'dialogical' expertise. The connotations of 'communication skills' – probably unfairly – still suggest some kind of 'transaction' between the different worlds of the professional and the service user.[2] There is some information to be shared or there is some distress to be acknowledged or empathy to be expressed. By contrast, what we have in mind includes the many different and more fundamental ways in which two (or more) individuals can both 'come together' and 'work together'. There are no formulas here and different respective roles will be appropriate in different kinds of circumstances and cases. But one way of understanding and indicating the potentially broad repertoire of possibilities is to think about the many different metaphors that can be and are applied to working together. Practitioners can be called upon both to help 'lead', and to 'follow' service users. They may help 'guide' or navigate their clients through services and experiences, and be guided by and responsive to them. They can be 'listeners' and 'learners', for example, attending to the immediate and wider predicaments of the people they are working with and, sometimes simultaneously, they can be 'educators'. They can be 'critical friends' part of the time, and 'advocates' part of the time. They should, of course, not assume that they have the only relevant expertise to bring to bear on the situation at hand. But, even where they do have special and necessary expertise, they can, at least in part, think of themselves as 'custodians' and 'curators' of that expertise

– finding ways of sharing it and opening it up to and for others
– rather than simply as the proprietors of it. This complexity
reflects that of individual identities as both hybrid and fluid.
As we discussed in chapter 5, even individuals do not occupy
a stable place in their relationship to services. They may be a
demanding 'consumer' in some respects and on some occasions, but in other circumstances they may feel the need, and
look to professionals to help them, to 'hand over' some of their
agency and invest their trust by adopting a more passive, even
compliant, role. Simple stories – either about 'paternalism' or
'equality' – and single snapshots of working relationships are
just misleading.

Relational expertise, including the flexibility to change
emphases in relationships according to circumstances, is a
crucial dimension of professionalism in an era where partnership has become an important value. It certainly cannot
and does not replace other forms of specialist knowledge and
capability, but it is increasingly recognized as a significant
component of the skill-set of even the most specialist and
technically focused practitioners.

Who are my exemplars?

We all learn from one another and, often without realizing it,
are influenced by the examples we come across. We may not
explicitly refer to our 'role models' – although many people
can easily be prompted to do so – but, nonetheless, we cannot
help but form our notion of what it means to do a good job, and
how to go about it, through the concrete instances we encounter. We will admire colleagues for a range of reasons. Some of
this may be because of their very developed specialized knowledge and practical skills. This is not to be underestimated. It
is very often what is most sought after by patients or service
users, but it will typically, as the last section indicated, also be
because of their 'personal style'. What we mean by this is the
way in which their character and personality is invested in,

and made manifest through, their work. There is all the difference in the world between admiring the way a robot does a job (which is something we can indeed watch with amazement on high-tech factory production lines) and admiring the way a person does a job. Everyone brings something different to their work, and it is a mistake to suppose that what they bring is 'superfluous', as if quality would necessarily be improved if everyone converged on exactly the same attitudes and behaviours (or, in other words, if they could be replaced with robots). Some degree of convergence in relation to elements of the content – the 'what' – of professional roles can be desirable (for example, in relation to key choices or techniques in surgery). This is part of the rationale of the evidence-based movement. But when it comes to the 'how' – to personal and professional styles – variation is arguably an added advantage. Indeed, from the point of view of wise resource allocation or the avoidance of waste, we could say that, unless institutions find ways of making space for, and benefiting from, people's characters and personalities, they will be failing to address something central.

Learning from our colleagues, and from others in general, is not straightforward. We might aspire to be like them in some respects but, in the end, we have to be ourselves. There is a limit to how much we can learn though simple imitation, although there is a place for this, especially in the early stages of a career when we are finding our way and trying to 'pass' in our roles. However, there is a deeper sense of imitation in which we might be inspired by the motives and commitments of colleagues and try to live up to these in our own way. It is likely that the colleagues we most admire will make an impression on us, and their work settings, through a broad-based set of capabilities and human qualities. In the end, perhaps the best lesson we can learn from them is the value of drawing upon our own humanity and using our own authentic resources, alongside the more generalizable elements of skill and knowledge.

However, this is much easier said than done. Work settings are not always nurturing and welcoming places and they can easily suffocate authenticity. In addition, they may marginalize, or even oppress, individuals with 'subaltern' or 'secondary' identities or value-sets. This applies, most notoriously, to people with the 'wrong' gender, sexual orientation, (dis)ability, class or 'race'. But it can also apply to individuals – whatever their social identity – who do not identify with the dominant, but often unofficial, norms of an organization. The latter can include such things as the way people tend to dress, talk to one another informally and in formal meetings, and the assumptions people make about what is important and not important. All of these things are manifest, for example, in the many discussions of gender in various work settings. But in all of these cases, debates about workplace norms and roles cannot be separated from questions about the politics of identity. For that reason, it is not uncommon for people to have as at least some of their real-world role models people who have found ways of making a contribution to, and being influential in, eroding narrow norms and in broadening horizons and visions against these kinds of odds.

Reflecting on exemplars is also a way of trying to identify and articulate the range of qualities or 'virtues' that are possible and can contribute towards filling a role successfully. These are the sorts of qualities that we try to collate together when we write character references for people. Although they are sometimes 'trotted out' without much thought, they indicate immensely valuable things. We might think of colleagues' dedication, determination, self-sacrifice, or their honesty, forthrightness, and courage, or perhaps their warmth, compassion, and gentleness and so on. If we are honest about ourselves, we are likely to think that we are personally more blessed with some of these qualities than we are with others. Of course, this exercise is also productive if we think – as we are perhaps more likely to – of the shortcomings, weaknesses or vices of our colleagues. Many of us are motivated by trying to avoid adopting some of the values, habits and attitudes of those we come into contact with!

Is professionalism a practical possibility for me?

Whether or not we identify with, or accept the label of, professionalism per se, we can all ask whether we can do a good job, and whether, in particular, we can use our 'licensed' knowledge and experience effectively. This is obviously partly a question about oneself – have I developed enough capability, confidence and experience? – but it is also a question about the conditions of one's work. As we have seen, there is a range of factors that can make professionalism more or less possible. These include the availability of suitable resources and the volume of work demanded, the models and practices of accountability in place, and, in particular, the scope for a degree of practitioner autonomy, where appropriate, to enable responsive and creative practice. Calling workers 'professionals', or deploying the value of 'professionalism' in the workplace is in itself beside the point. Indeed, as Evetts[3] underlines, the use of the language and ideology of professionalism is, on some occasions, best understood as a device to strengthen the managerial control, and effectively inhibit the freedom of manoeuvre, of a workforce.

In practice, we are liable to feel that we have to give a compound answer to any question about the scope of our autonomy. Work is not monolithic. In some of our tasks, we may feel we have the necessary leeway to use our expertise properly, whilst in others we may judge that we are frustrated in damaging ways. Similarly, there can be substantial variations between services and settings, or between pockets and 'micro-climates' in the same services – with different kinds and degrees of team-working, support, licence and trust available to us. Even if we judge that we are generally constrained and inhibited from using our expertise appropriately, there are still ways in which we can do our best in difficult circumstances – by attempting to challenge the prevailing climate and by limiting, as far as possible, the negative consequences of the models we are being asked to adhere to. (The first is, on our account, an attempt to assert professionalism and the latter an attempt to hold onto vestiges of professionalism.)

But one thing is clear. There is comparatively little we can do solely as individuals to make professionalism possible. Professionalism is, in essence, a 'team sport', a social phenomenon. The kinds of expertise and functions that identify groups of practitioners in health and social care are developed, recognized, transmitted and critically questioned through social and collective processes. It is possible to be an unusual, eccentric, or even maverick, practitioner but there are limits to the degree of eccentricity that is possible whilst remaining recognizable as a member of a particular professional group. This means that individuals who feel that they are either not granted the freedom of manoeuvre or the structural support to do a good job need to work collectively to try and change things. If they are not simply to leave their role (which may be an option where they feel they can make more of a difference in some other way, of course), they will need to embrace the politics of their profession in some way. This might be through engagement in the official and collegial processes of their professional body, for example helping to define standards and campaign for changes in regulations and governance. It might be through the micro-politics of their employing organizations, or through disputes with employers at a national level over terms and conditions of work. It might be as part of some broader social and political movements engaged in parliamentary lobbying or extra-parliamentary activism. Whether or not this is always overtly signalled, professions, and the conditions of professionalism, are political matters. Indeed, as has been understood, at least since it was articulated by Aristotle, human beings are inherently social and political creatures. Professionalism depends upon at least some members of professional groups embracing this fact.

How can I handle dilemmas and routine moral stress?

Engaging with the micro-politics of the workplace is only one, albeit important, example of the many challenges practitioners face. All of life, including our work life, can be seen as an exercise in 'resource allocation' where we are the resource we are attempting to allocate. What ought I to be paying attention to, what ought I to be channelling my energies towards, which battles should I be fighting, or where or when should I be engaged in peace-making? One pervasive dilemma is how to divide our time, attention and efforts between, on the one hand, getting on with the immediate demands of our role and, on the other hand, helping to secure or change our 'role environment' – the institutional policies, structures and cultures that we work within. Different individuals will have different combinations of interests, dispositions, capacities and opportunities in this regard.

There is no one 'right' balance here. Partly this is a practical question. The sheer intensity of some jobs and the relative inflexibility and intractability of some workplace systems means that only the most dynamic, resilient and self-confident (or well-supported) individuals can find the tenacity to help question and shape their role environment. Partly it is a genuine ethical dilemma. There are often good arguments for 'accepting your lot', embracing and inhabiting your professional role, and getting on with doing the best job possible. But there are also good arguments for resisting norms that seem to be damaging your workplace, or for standing back from and critically questioning your role and the things you are expected to do. Is it better to be more focused and effective in doing something you regard as sub-optimal, or to try and improve things when you may not succeed, may even be mistaken in thinking you 'know better', and may dissipate your energies as a result?[4] Obviously, it will vary from case to case, but the whole point about dilemmas is that there is no formulaic way of working out the best answer in advance, or of knowing which sort of case you are dealing with. It is a matter of making a series of difficult ongoing judgements.

Of course, the dilemmas that practitioners face, and are entangled with, are not all about the correct orientation to their professional role. Indeed, quite rightly, most of the ethical tensions and dilemmas discussed under the heading of 'professional ethics' are not so self-referential but are about balancing the competing values and interests of other people – not least the service users and publics being served. It is not possible, nor would it make sense, to review all of these dilemmas here. But it may be worth a brief final reminder as to how diverse, complex, deep-seated and 'routine' these are. Practitioners are permanently having to balance the 'wants' and welfare of each individual, the interests and perspectives of individuals with those of family members, groups and the wider society, the competing needs of different service users and the demands and expectations of service users, employing organizations and other agencies, including professional bodies. And, in every case, these ethical tensions are bound up with technical and pragmatic judgements and made in the context of considerable institutional constraints. These incredibly challenging balancing acts are close to the heart of professionalism. They depend upon practitioners' accumulated knowledge and experience and, indeed, handling them is itself a key part of the expertise that is 'licensed' in professional roles.

Some analysts have used the label 'moral distress'[5] to capture the consequences of living with these competing demands. Practitioners cannot do all the things they might like to and cannot satisfactorily address the legitimate concerns of every relevant party – and, crucially, they could not do so even with infinite effort and resources because dilemmas pull us in different directions. This does not only apply to large or dramatic ethical dilemmas (for example, whether or not to turn a life-support machine off, or whether or not to recommend

someone is taken into care or institutionalized) but to countless everyday decisions. Nor are we necessarily conscious of
being 'distressed' by these balancing acts. The pressures they
put us under may often fall below the radar of our consciousness but are nonetheless real. For that reason, we find the
notion of 'routine moral stress' a useful one here.[6] This is a different phenomenon to the costs of 'emotional labour' and the
associated risks of 'burn-out', although it overlaps with this. In
both cases, what is highlighted is the way in which the whole
person of the practitioner is implicated in her or his work. Both
'ethical labour' and 'emotional labour' – the former relating
to the burden of determining what is for the best, all things
considered, and the latter the burden of managing one's own
and others' feelings in one's job – call upon the character and
'human' resource of practitioners. They overlap because ethics
and emotions inform one another.

Is my role a mask for vice or a scaffold for virtue?

In chapter 1, we explored – using extreme cases – the possibility that professional roles can serve both as a mask for vice
and as a scaffold for virtue. Of course, individuals only occupy
roles; they are not wholly defined by them. This opens up the
question of how roles serve individuals. To occupy a professional role is to receive a certain kind of social legitimacy and
status. In a few cases, this is symbolized by the entitlement
to wear certain kinds of clothing or uniform (for example, as
is the case with some nurses or barristers). But this notion
can also be extended metaphorically – to be granted professional status is to have one's idiosyncratic history and identity
clothed in something uniform and respectable. In a professional role, one shares an official identity that carries a range
of symbolic messages – messages of reassurance, trustworthi-
ness and capability. Such 'clothing' can be perceived as a mask
in productive ways. For example, for people who are adjusting

to their roles and responsibilities, it can help conceal feelings of inadequacy and thereby support confidence. (Even in these positive cases, though, we need to be mindful of the danger that adherence to official role identities and norms can inhibit individuals from making their full humanity available in their work.) However, the clothing of legitimacy carries a considerable risk that we hide behind our roles in more worrying ways: that we use our roles to cover up laziness, pettiness, selfishness or even worse faults. The more power and status we have, by definition the greater the opportunities and temptations to succumb to these forms of disguise. Someone who is deeply cynical could represent high-status social roles, including some professional roles, as nothing more than a mechanism for clothing imperfect human beings in the guise of automatic respectability.

By contrast, and this is the possibility we wish to emphasize, professional roles can be seen as providing an engine for good ends. They enable individuals to take on important social responsibilities, and they provide communities of practice and the collegial and critical scrutiny of others. In so doing, they can help individuals feel that they are in a position, and have the resources, to do things that they would feel unable to undertake otherwise. Over time, they can help individuals cultivate the personal dispositions and the networks of support that make them ever more energetic and bold in their efforts to support and care for other people. Of course, these two readings – the cynical and the idealistic – are not completely incompatible. As we have noted in several places, identities are hybrid and ambivalence is often a wise attitude to adopt in our appraisal of motives and practices. It is certainly crucial when we reflect on our own motives and practices. Reflective practice must include the capacity to question the legitimating stories we tell ourselves. At minimum, this means we should not assume that we are simply 'doing good' but be ready to critically examine the ethical ambiguities that attach to our roles and activities. Achieving this critical distance is very important but it is also very demanding. This is because professional roles have powerful effects on role holders: they shape practitioner's self-understandings and ethical sensibilities, and this means that certain purposes and priorities become 'taken for granted'. Without being open to critique from and dialogue with others, it is very difficult to 'stand back' from one's own frame of reference.

Although we have underlined the stresses of occupying a professional role in health and social care, these stresses are, of course, only part of the picture. Many of the things that people do are chosen because they are both challenging and fulfilling and, more particularly, because the challenge is what makes them fulfilling. Anyone who practises a musical instrument, trains for a half-marathon, or even just sets out to cook an elaborate meal for friends knows this to be true. Stretching and testing ourselves is central to the possibility of fulfilment and can – although, of course, not in every moment – be enjoyable too. There is no reason why these things cannot also apply in the world of work. Indeed, perhaps the best way of distinguishing between desirable and undesirable jobs is by asking whether or not the roles provide these opportunities for fulfilment and enjoyment. It sounds very 'worthy' to talk about acquiring the intellectual, civic, ethical and emotional virtues and know-how needed to be an excellent health or social care practitioner. But another way of looking at developing these personal qualities that underpin the exercise of professionalism is to see it as a privilege to be able to learn, and to find satisfaction and sometimes even fun, whilst doing one's job.

Conclusion

We have suggested that professionalism, as the accomplished exercise of expertise-based social authority, is still a fundamentally important social value. This very broad concept of professionalism has relevance to the many new and emerging occupational roles in health and social care, as well as to what

were historically thought of as the traditional professions.
Changing social and political conditions and cultural mores,
however, mean that traditional role expectations have had to be
rethought for all professional roles and that the accompanying
'value-set' of professionalism has changed. It is impossible to
think of professionals as 'special' in the same sense that they
once were. We live in times where there is widespread scepticism about both expertise and social authority, and where
people are less ready to defer to, or accept, paternalistic pre-
scriptions. Expertise and authority take more diffused and
negotiated forms. There is also much more sensitivity to, and
reflexivity about, the ethical ambiguity of social practices – it is
not only critical sociology but also popular opinion that would
hesitate to attribute unqualified altruism to any group of workers. Yet, despite this scepticism, people do look to health and
social care professionals for help and support, and do so need-
ing to be able to place trust in them. There is as much need
for professionalism as ever there was. New conditions of professionalism are thus peculiarly challenging. Practitioners
need to be able to work both with service users and for them.
At the same time, they are required to be mindful of competing kinds of accountability – not just narrow institutional
accountability but also their accountability to populations
(for example, through system or public health ends), as well
as their accountability to the person or group directly in front
of them. The routine dilemmas generated by these balancing
acts are fraught with difficulty. Professionals may no longer
be encouraged to think of themselves as individually special,
but they are certainly placed in very special positions and it is
arguable that the dispositions that are needed to succeed in
these positions are 'extra-special'.

To adopt a professional role in health or social care is in
many cases to take up a considerable ethical and emotional
burden and at the same time to get the opportunity and social
permission to use one's knowledge and capabilities to make
a contribution to other people's well-being. Whatever formal

systems of accountability are in place, there is no avoiding personal accountability for one's actual and potential contribution. However, it is, of course, important that individual practitioners are not left to cope alone but are supported both formally and informally by colleagues (and ideally by others, too). It is to be hoped that the official structures and mechanisms provided by professional bodies and employers offer much of this necessary support and guidance. With luck, one also has good colleagues close by with whom one can, at least, complain about the inadequacy of official structures and dream and scheme about how to make things better and with whom one can celebrate survival and successes. Given these conditions and forms of support, it makes sense to aspire to do a good job and even to pursue ideals in everyday practice.

Notes

CHAPTER 1   HEROES AND ANTI-HEROES

1 Brian Hurwitz, 'Healthcare Serial Killings: Was the Case of Dr Harold Shipman Unthinkable?' in *Bioethics, Medicine and the Criminal Law: Medicine, Crime and Society, Vol. 2,* ed. Danielle Griffiths and Andrew Sanders (Cambridge: Cambridge University Press, 2013), 13–42.
2 Craig Webber, *Psychology and Crime* (London: Sage, 2009).
3 Idealistic readings – such as ones you might see in the publicity material for a professional body – are those that treat professions simply as a force for good and assert or assume we can place our trust in professionals. Idealistic readings tend to stress values such as altruism and the public interest. Critical readings – such as ones you might see in certain sociological analyses or in campaigning material from aggrieved client groups – question the contributions made by professions and professionals and invite awareness, and suspicion, of professional power. Critical readings often stress the anti-democratic and anti-egalitarian tendencies of professions.
4 Clearly, this inside–outside distinction is a very crude one. Practitioners who see their work through a social lens, for example a Marxist or communitarian-conservative lens, will have an inside perspective that attempts to incorporate what we are calling an outside perspective.
5 Pierre Bourdieu and Jean-Claude Passeron, *Reproduction in Education, Society and Culture* (London and Beverly Hills: Sage, 1977).
6 See, for example, Deborah Lupton, *The Imperative of Health: Public Health and the Regulated Body* (London: Sage, 1995) and Robin Bunton and Alan Petersen, *Foucault, Health and Medicine* (Abingdon: Routledge, 1997).
7 Susan Hinze, 'Gender and the Body of Medicine or at Least Some Body Parts: (Re)constructing the Prestige Hierarchy

of Medical Specialities', *The Sociological Quarterly* 40 (March 1999): 217–39; Heidi Lempp and Alan Cribb, 'The Diversity and Unity of the Hidden Curriculum: Medical Knowledge in an Era of Personalised Healthcare', in *The Hidden Curriculum and Health Professions Education*, ed. Fred Hafferty and Joseph O'Donnell (Hanover, New Hampshire: Dartmouth College Press, 2014).

CHAPTER 2   VARIETIES OF PROFESSIONALISM

1 Walter Bryce Gallie, 'Essentially Contested Concepts', *Proceedings of the Aristotelian Society* 56 (1956): 167–98.
2 George Ritzer, *Encyclopedia of Social Theory* (London: Sage, 2004), 603.
3 Daryl Koehn, *The Ground of Professional Ethics* (London and New York: Routledge, 1994), 56.
4 Talcott Parsons, 'The Professions and Social Structure', *Social Forces* 17 (May 1939): 457–67.
5 Emile Durkheim, *Professional Ethics and Civic Morals* (London and New York: Routledge, 2003).
6 Terence James Johnson, *Professions and Power* (London: Macmillan, 1972).
7 Magali Sarfatti Larson, *The Rise of Professionalism: A Sociological Analysis* (Berkeley, Los Angeles and London: University of California Press, 1977).
8 Johnson, *Professions and Power*, 45.
9 Larson, *Rise of Professionalism*, xvii.
10 For example, Amitai Etzioni (ed.), *The Semi-Professions and their Organization: Teachers, Nurses, Social Workers* (New York: The Free Press, 1969).
11 Abraham Flexner, 'Is Social Work a Profession?' *School and Society* 1 (June 1915): 901–11.
12 Royal College of Physicians, *Doctors in Society: Medical Professionalism in a Changing World* (London: RCP, 2005), 16.
13 In the account of professionalism we offer in the second half of this book, we make use of the language of 'authority'. Whilst strongly agreeing with the implications of this RCP report that ideas such as mastery, control and superiority are outdated and unhelpful, we would argue that the notion of authority needs to be disentangled from these other ideas. Authority does have some unfortunate connotations but we think it is better, and

more honest, to retain some focus on the notion of authority (and for that matter power too) when analysing the values of professionalism.

14 Bruce G. Robinson and Peter M. Brooks, 'The Medical Workforce of the Future', *MJA Open* 1 Supp. l3, (July 2012): 4.

15 Adrian Edwards and Glyn Elwyn (eds), *Shared Decision-Making in Health Care* (Oxford: Oxford University Press, 2009); 'Salzburg Statement on Shared Decision-Making', *British Medical Journal* 342 (March 2011): d1745.

16 See, for example: Rob Horne, *Concordance, Adherence and Compliance in Medicine Taking. Report for the National Coordinating Centre for NHS Service Delivery and Organisation (NCCSDO)* (London: NCCSDO, 2005); Royal Pharmaceutical Society of Great Britain (RPSGB), *From Compliance to Concordance* (London: RPSGB, 1997); and Jane Askham and Alison Chisholm, *Patient-Centred Medical Professionalism* (Oxford: Picker Institute, 2006).

17 Julia Evetts, 'A New Professionalism? Challenges and Opportunities', *Current Sociology* 59 (July 2011): 406–22.

18 At least, this applies in any system that depends upon 'pooled resources', for example, in the UK NHS or any 'single-payer' system or social or private insurance scheme. This need not apply in a simple fee-for-service private model.

19 It is worth noting that this aspect of new professionalism – the trajectory towards 'partnership working' – which we have been citing in this chapter assumes the background of a particular kind of developed welfare economy and a history of embedded 'top-down' assumptions about professionalism. There is no reason to assume that the same transitions happen in the same way and stage in all global settings. Indeed, reviews of 'cutting edge' innovations in partnership-working often cite examples from developing economies, e.g. Erik Rasmussen, Kalle Jørgensen and Stephen Leyshon (eds), *Person-Centred Care: Co-Creating a Healthcare Sector for the Future* (DNV GL and Monday Morning/Sustainia, 2014), http://www.sustainia.me/resources/publications/Person-Centred_Healthcare.pdf.

CHAPTER 3   IMPOSSIBLE DREAMS

1 Daryl Koehn, *The Ground of Professional Ethics* (London and New York: Routledge, 1994).

2 Marie Haug and Marvin Sussman, 'Professional Autonomy and the Revolt of the Client', *Social Problems* 17 (Autumn 1969): 153–61.
3 Michaela Pfadenhauer, 'Crisis or Decline? Problems of Legitimation and Loss of Trust in Modern Professionalism', *Current Sociology* 54 (July 2006): 573.
4 Frederic Hafferty and Brian Castellani, 'The Increasing Complexities of Professionalism', *Academic Medicine* 85 (February 2010): 288–301.
5 See, for example, Lucien Leap Institute, National Patient Safety Foundation, *Through the Eyes of the Workforce: Creating Joy, Meaning and Safer Health Care* (Boston, MA: National Patient Safety Foundation, 2013); and Point of Care Foundation, *How to Engage Staff in the NHS and Why it Matters* (London: Point of Care Foundation, 2014).
6 This has been recognized, for example, in debates about whether nursing should be thought of as a profession at all or whether it is better to think of it as a 'managed occupation' or perhaps as a semi-profession.
7 See, for example, John Clarke, Sharon Gewirtz and Eugene McLaughlin (eds), *New Managerialism, New Welfare* (London: Sage, 2000); Jane Green, *Education, Professionalism and the Quest for Accountability: Hitting the target but missing the point* (London: Routledge, 2011); Steve Rogowski, 'Managers, Managerialism and Social Work with Children and Families: The Deformation of a Profession?', *Practice* 23 (May 2011): 157–67; and Marilyn M. Rosenthal, 'Medical Professional Autonomy in an era of Accountability and Regulation: Voices of Doctors under Siege', in *Managing Professional Identities: Knowledge, Performativity and the New Professional*, ed. Mike Dent and Stephen Whitehead (London: Routledge, 2013).
8 Although it is not always appreciated, the need to find a balance between statistical generalization and particular judgements oriented towards and by individuals was actually recognized by (and 'contained' within) Sackett et al.'s (1996) original and influential definition of evidence-based medicine as 'the conscientious, explicit and judicious use of current best evidence in making decisions about the care of individual patients. The practice of evidence-based medicine means integrating individual clinical expertise with the best available external clinical evidence from systematic research.' David L. Sackett, William M. C. Rosenberg, J. A. Muir Gray, R. Brian Haynes and

W. Scott Richardson, 'Evidence-Based Medicine: What It is and
What It isn't', *British Medical Journal* 312 (January 1996): 71–2.

9 Haug and Sussman, 'Professional Autonomy', 153–61.

10 It is even possible to suggest – even though this sounds
paradoxical – that this process of co-option represents a
'professionalization project'. On this account, lay expertise is at
least in part being professionalized.

11 For example, versions of them can be presented as
strengthening democratic conceptions of professionalism, or
versions of them can be combined with market conceptions of
professionalism.

CHAPTER 4   LICENSED TO CARE

1 Susan Wolf, *Meaning in Life and Why it Matters* (Princeton:
Princeton University Press, 2012).

2 Helen's exact job title is probably confined to the United
Kingdom where she works, but there are many analogous roles
in other health systems such as 'hospital-based outreach' or
'liaison' nursing. More specifically, Helen's role falls under
the heading of 'Advanced Practice Oncology Nursing' and is
undertaken by someone who is a 'specialist' or 'advanced' nurse
practitioner and who has undergone higher-level education,
including training in clinical duties such as prescribing.

3 Eliot Freidson, *Professionalism: The Third Logic* (Chicago:
Chicago University Press, 2001).

4 Gilbert Ryle, 'Knowing How and Knowing That: The
Presidential Address', *Proceedings of the Aristotelian Society New
Series* 46 (1945–6): 1–16.

5 Richard Stanley Peters, *Ethics and Education* (London: Allen and
Unwin, 1966).

6 A notable exception to this influential stream of 'value-
neutral' approaches to professionalism is the 'values-based
medicine' or 'values-based practice' approach to theory and
practice, originated by Professor Bill Fulford, which has made
some significant inroads into clinical education and which
unapologetically places the values of health care centre-stage (as
a necessary complement to evidence and EBM). See, for example,
Bill Fulford, Ed Peile and Heidi Carroll, *Essential Values-Based
Practice: Clinical Stories Linking Values with People* (Cambridge,
UK: Cambridge University Press, 2012).

7 Isabel Menzies Lyth, 'The Functions of Social Systems as a Defence Against Anxiety: A Report on a Study of the Nursing Service of a General Hospital', *Human Relations* 13 (1959): 95–121.

8 Sarah Bignold and Alan Cribb, 'Towards the Reflexive Medical School: The Hidden Curriculum and Medical Education Research', *Studies in Higher Education* 24 (June 1999): 195–209.

9 Nicky James, 'Care = Organisation + Physical Labour + Emotional Labour', *Sociology of Health and Illness* 14(4) (2008): 489–509; Eric Larson and Xin Yao, 'Clinical Empathy as Emotional Labor in the Patient–Physician Relationship', *Journal of the American Medical Association* 293 (March 2005): 1100–6.

CHAPTER 5   INTEGRITY AT WORK

1 John Clarke and Janet Newman, 'Elusive Publics: Knowledge, Power and Public Service Reform', in *Changing Teacher Professionalism: International Trends, Challenges and Ways Forward*, ed. Sharon Gewirtz, Pat Mahony, Ian Hextall and Alan Cribb (London: Routledge, 2009), 48.

2 Tom Beauchamp and James Childress, *Principles of Biomedical Ethics*, 6th edn (Oxford: Oxford University Press, 2009).

3 Health visitors, in the UK context, are specialized community nurses who offer support to families from the time of pregnancy and through early childhood in a variety of care settings, including the home.

4 Julie Catherine Greenway, Vikki Ann Entwistle and Ruud ter Meulen, 'Ethical Tensions Associated with the Promotion of Public Health Policy in Health Visiting: A Qualitative Investigation of Health Visitors' Views', *Primary Health Care Research & Development* 14 (April 2013): 200–11.

5 Janine Jolly, *The National Teenage Pregnancy Strategy: A Qualitative Exploration of a Public Health Policy*, unpublished PhD thesis (London: King's College London, 2011).

6 Sarah Banks, *Ethics and Values in Social Work*, 3rd edn (Basingstoke: Palgrave Macmillan, 2006).

7 Alan Cribb, 'Integrity at Work: Managing Routine Moral Stress in Professional Roles', *Nursing Philosophy* 12(2) (April 2011): 119–27.

8 The *Ethics in Social Work, Statement of Principles* jointly issued in 2004 by the International Federation of Social Workers

(IFSW) and the International Association of Schools of Social Work (IASSW), for example, includes a whole section on social justice which differentiates between five facets, in summary: challenging discrimination, recognizing diversity, distributing resources equitably, challenging unjust policies and practices, and working in solidarity. IFSW and IASSW, *Ethics in Social Work, Statement of Principles* (Bern: IFSW and IASSW, 2004).

9 The fact that many patient organizations, including umbrella organizations such as National Voices in England and its equivalent in other countries, exercise a degree of collective autonomy and have an independent voice which is granted legitimacy by senior policy makers and others is an argument for viewing them in some ways as analogous to professional organizations. However, some of the other characteristics of professions and professionalism (for example, the socially sanctioned and demanded accountability of individual members in relation to specific roles) fit them much less neatly.

10 IFSW and IASSW, *Ethics in Social Work, Statement of Principles*.

11 This is just a specific case of a fundamental conundrum arising from the relationship between identity and freedom, which is analysed in Sartre's existentialism – that is, whether we imagine ourselves to be 'identical' with our roles (the 'error of facticity') or 'independent' of our roles (the 'error of transcendence'). Jean-Paul Sartre, *Being and Nothingness* (New York: Philosophical Library, 1948).

12 Michael Lipsky, *Street-Level Bureaucracy: Dilemmas of the Individual in Public Services* (New York: Russell Sage Foundation, 2010).

CHAPTER 6   SUPPORTING PROFESSIONALISM

1 Jane Broadbent and Richard Laughlin, '"Accounting Logic" and Controlling Professionals', in *The End of the Professions? The Restructuring of Professional Work*, ed. Jane Broadbent, Michael Dietrich and Jennifer Roberts (Abingdon: Routledge, 2005), 33–48.

2 Elements of this example are drawn from the empirical work of our colleague, Andrew Papanikitas. See Andrew Papanikitas, *From the Classroom to the Clinic: Ethics, Education and General Practice*, unpublished PhD Thesis (London: King's College London, 2014).

3 Many educational experiences combine different elements and there are strong parallels between formal education provision and informal in-service education. In the example discussed here, Lauren might have been a GP in training or even an undergraduate medical student. In each case, she could have raised broadly similar concerns with Angela and there might have been closely analogous opportunities for teaching and learning. The differences relate partly to the degree of immersion in and engagement with the professional dilemmas under consideration. There are both emotional and ethical differences between (a) exploring the issues 'academically' as someone who is imaginatively considering the role position of a GP, compared either with (b) someone who is learning and adjusting to the role in a way that is recognized as provisional and accompanied by structured support, or with (c) someone who is actually occupying the role with all the attendant responsibilities and accountabilities.

4 Chris Argyris and Donald A. Schön, *Organizational Learning II: Theory, Method and Practice* (Reading, MA: Addison-Wesley, 1996); Mark Easterby-Smith and Luis Araujo, *Organizational Learning and the Learning Organization: Developments in Theory and Practice* (London: Sage, 1999).

5 Heather Hodkinson, 'Improving Schoolteachers' Workplace Learning', in *Changing Teacher Professionalism: International Trends, Challenges and Ways Forward*, ed. Sharon Gewirtz, Pat Mahony, Ian Hextall and Alan Cribb (Abingdon: Routledge, 2009), 157–69. See also the literatures on continuing professional development and communities of practice (e.g. Paul Hager, 'Current Theories of Workplace Learning: A Critical Assessment', in *International Handbook of Educational Policy* (Part Two), ed. Nina Bascia, Alister Cumming, Amanda Datnow, Kenneth Leithwood and David Livingstone (Dordrecht: Springer, 2005), 829–46; and Jean Lave and Etienne Wenger, *Situated Learning: Legitimate Peripheral Participation* (Cambridge: Cambridge University Press, 1991).

6 See, for example, the NHS Leadership Academy and its Leadership Framework, http://www.leadershipacademy.nhs.uk/discover/leadership-framework/

7 Craig Pearce and Henry Sims, 'Shared Leadership: Toward a Multi-level Theory of Leadership', *Advances in Interdisciplinary Studies of Work Teams* 7 (2001): 115–39; Richard Bolden, 'Distributed Leadership in Organizations: A Review of Theory

and Research', *International Journal of Management Reviews* 13 (September 2011): 251–69.

8 See, for example, Onora O'Neill, *A Question of Trust, The BBC Reith Lectures 2002* (Cambridge: Cambridge University Press, 2002); and John Roberts, 'No One is Perfect: The Limits of Transparency and an Ethic for "Intelligent" Accountability', *Accounting, Organizations and Society* 34 (November 2009): 957–70.

9 Donald Schön, *The Reflective Practitioner: How Professionals Think in Action* (Aldershot: Ashgate, 1995), 338.

10 Hodkinson, 'Improving Schoolteachers' Workplace Learning'.

CHAPTER 7   PROFESSIONAL IDENTITIES

1 See William F. May, *Beleaguered Rulers: The Public Obligation of the Professional* (Louisville, Kentucky: Westminster John Knox Press, 1995).

2 Valerie Iles, *Why Reforming the NHS Doesn't Work: The Importance of Understanding How Good People Offer Bad Care* (Really Learning, 2011). http://www.reallylearning.com/Free_Resources/Really_Managing_Healthcare/reforming.pdf

3 Julia Evetts, 'A New Professionalism? Challenges and Opportunities', *Current Sociology* 59 (July 2011).

4 Julia Annas, 'My Station and its Duties: Ideals and the Social Embeddedness of Virtue', *Proceedings of the Aristotelian Society* (January 2002): 109–23.

5 M. L. Raines, 'Ethical Decision Making in Nurses', *Jona's Healthcare Law, Ethics and Regulation* 2 (March 2000): 29–41; S. Kalvemark, A. Hoglun, M. Hansson, P. Westerholm and B. Arnetz, 'Living with Conflicts – Ethical Dilemmas and Moral Distress in the Health Care System', *Social Science & Medicine* 58 (March 2004): 1075–84.

6 Alan Cribb, 'Integrity at Work: Managing Routine Moral Stress in Professional Roles', *Nursing Philosophy* 12(2) (April 2011).

Index

Index compiled by Frank Pert